Body Care

**Also in the Growing, Growing Strong:
A Whole Health Curriculum for Young Children Series**

Fitness and Nutrition

Safety

Social and Emotional Well-Being

Community and Environment

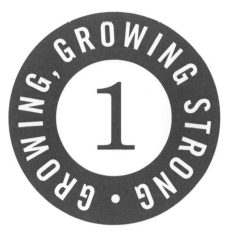

GROWING, GROWING STRONG

1

A Whole Health Curriculum for Young Children

Body Care

Third Edition

Connie Jo Smith

Charlotte M. Hendricks

Becky S. Bennett

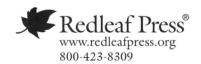

Redleaf Press®
www.redleafpress.org
800-423-8309

Published by Redleaf Press
10 Yorkton Court
St. Paul, MN 55117
www.redleafpress.org

First edition published 1997. Second edition 2006. Third edition 2014.
Cover design by Jim Handrigan
Cover photograph © Ocean Photography/Veer
Interior design by Percolator
Typeset in Stone Informal, Matrix Script, and Trade Gothic
Illustrations by Chris Wold Dyrud
Photograph on page 58 © Ocean Photography/Veer
Printed in the United States of America
20 19 18 17 16 15 14 13   1 2 3 4 5 6 7 8

Library of Congress Cataloging-in-Publication Data
Smith, Connie Jo.
    Body care / Connie Jo Smith, Charlotte M. Hendricks, and Becky S. Bennett. — Third edition.
       pages cm — (Growing, growing strong: a whole health curriculum for young children)
    Revision of: Growing, growing strong: a whole health curriculum for young children.
    ISBN 978-1-60554-240-9 (pbk. : alk. paper)
    ISBN 978-1-60554-331-4 (e-book)
    1. Health education (Preschool)—United States. 2. Health education (Elementary)—United States.
    3. Curriculum planning—United States.   I. Hendricks, Charlotte M. 1957- II. Bennett, Becky S., 1954- III. Title.
    LB1140.5.H4S64 2014
    372.37—dc23
                                                                                    2013017165

Printed on acid-free paper

To the memory of my parents, Nevolyn and George. My mother taught me that a sense of humor is an essential life skill, regardless of age. My dad taught me the importance of love and independence.

—Connie Jo

To Gayle Cunningham for guidance and friendship, and to Don Palmer for always being there for me. And in memory of Nic Frising for showing the humor in life through art.

—Charlotte

To the memory of my parents, Charlie and Jeanette, who gave me life, love, and encouragement to follow my dreams. And to my partner, Connie, who has taught me so much about the early care and education field, love, and family.

—Becky

Contents

Acknowledgments

We would like to express heartfelt appreciation to our talented, hardworking, and ever-positive editor, Kyra Ostendorf. This book is much richer for her ideas, guidance, and smiles—those given in person and those arriving through electronic communication ;-). Thanks to Elena Fultz and Grace Fowler, interns at Redleaf Press, who assisted in technical editing. We are grateful to David Heath for his initial editing support and encouragement. And, of course, we want to acknowledge all the individuals we have had professional encounters with over the years, as each contact has helped us grow and has enhanced our work.

Introduction

As young children become aware of their body parts and start to understand how the parts work individually and together, they can begin to appreciate and accept responsibility for their bodies and their health. Though parents, caregivers, and other adults are primarily responsible for children's health and safety, young children can begin to nurture lifelong habits that will greatly affect their quality of life. This curriculum introduces positive body care habits.

Children are naturally curious about their body parts, especially the external body parts that are visible. They also recognize differences in their bodies, such as in height, weight, skin color, and physical ability. Begin teaching children about their bodies by identifying external body parts (for example, eyes, ears, nose, tongue, and fingers) and associating them with specific functions. Use the five senses to introduce how specific body parts work. Through hands-on activities like those provided in this book, children can explore how these body parts work together.

Preschool children will not and do not need to understand how diseases are spread (such as through direct contact, airborne transmission, and consumption of food and beverages), and the concept of invisible germs is usually beyond their comprehension. But teachers can help children begin to recognize that their actions may affect their health. Teachers should model and encourage routine health activities, including hand washing, coughing or sneezing into the elbow, and toothbrushing. With instruction, modeling, and practice, teachers can help children begin to develop self-help skills, an ability to respond to their body cues, and decision-making skills, which all can impact their health.

Topics in this curriculum include recognizing body parts, understanding the five senses, washing hands and practicing good hygiene, brushing teeth and promoting good oral health, avoiding germs, and taking medicine. The activities and resources will help children learn ways to feel good about themselves and their bodies, prevent the spread of diseases, and gain a measure of independence and control in their lives.

Each chapter covers one topic and starts with an overview that includes suggested interest area materials, learning objectives, vocabulary words to introduce and use (which should include vocabulary words in the languages spoken by the families of children in the class), supports for creating the learning environment, and suggestions for evaluating children's understanding of the topic. The overview is followed by activity ideas. To identify the areas of development and learning integrated into the activity, icons appear with each one:

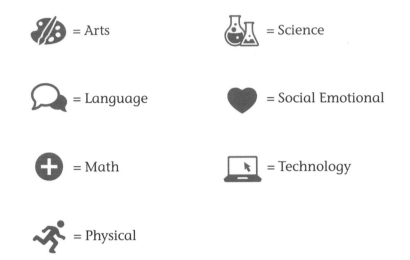

= Arts

= Science

= Language

= Social Emotional

= Math

= Technology

= Physical

Each chapter concludes with a family information page and a take-home family activity page, both of which can be photocopied from the book and distributed to families. These pages can also be downloaded from the Growing, Growing Strong page at www.redleafpress.org for electronic sharing or printing.

INTEREST AREA MATERIALS

Dramatic Play

multiethnic dolls and toy people with different body types and hair types, including some with teeth

adaptive equipment for dolls and toy people, such as wheelchairs, crutches, glasses, and hearing aids

sunglasses and hats

kneepads, wrist pads, and helmets

eyeglass frames and eye patches

eye chart

herbs and spices

fabric of various sizes and textures

baby bathtub or dishpan

empty shampoo and conditioner containers

ribbons, scarves, bows, and barrettes

hair dryer (without the cord)

empty toothpaste containers

clothesline and clothespins

bath toys

shoes and shoeshine brushes

ice packs

empty hot-water bottle

nonbreakable full-body mirrors and hand mirrors

Blocks

goggles

helmets

hard hats

work gloves

wooden animals

multiethnic wooden people with different physical abilities

tape measures

shoe boxes and hatboxes for building

washcloths to incorporate into buildings

hair rollers for building and hauling

empty shampoo containers for building and hauling

empty toothpaste containers and soap cartons for building and hauling

empty medicine bottles and lids for building and hauling

Table Toys

dollhouse with multiethnic dolls or toy people

puzzles of multiethnic people

knob and jigsaw puzzles of body parts

paper dolls with protective clothing

lotto games that include body parts

pattern games and cards

tactile matching puzzles and games

grab bag with textured objects

lacing cards

empty medicine bottles and lids for matching

tweezers and cotton balls for filling and emptying containers

Art

skull and skeleton artwork

paper of various colors and kinds (tracing, tissue, aluminum foil, cellophane, gummed, origami, fingerpaint, metallic, carbon, typing, and drawing)

glue in a variety of colors

skin-tone colors of paint, crayons, markers, pencils, and modeling clay

string

sand

food coloring

cloth

ribbon

supplies for visual and cultural variety

fingerpaints

materials for hand models, such as clay, Styrofoam, papier-mâché supplies, and short pieces of vinyl-covered wire

wig-making supplies, such as yarn, string, shower caps, and swim caps

paintbrushes, vegetable brushes, toothbrushes, and hairbrushes

new unused syringes without needles for painting

spray bottles for painting

Language Arts

finger and hand puppets

multiethnic hairstyle magazines that
    include diverse styles

sewing patterns

clothing catalogs

luggage tags

photographs of teeth

prescription pads

Library

All the Colors We Are by Katie Kissinger

The Dirty Little Boy by Margaret Wise
    Brown

From Head to Toe by Eric Carle

It's Okay to Be Different by Todd Parr

My Five Senses by Aliki

*Those Mean Nasty Dirty Downright
    Disgusting but . . . Invisible Germs*
    by Judith Anne Rice

*Throw Your Tooth on the Roof: Tooth
    Traditions from Around the World*
    by Selby B. Beeler

Science and Math

dolls or toy people that can be
    taken apart

charts and posters of the body

X-rays of the body

X-rays of teeth that show roots

tape measures

weight scales (digital and analog)

skeleton models and illustrations

kaleidoscopes

sanitized bones (chicken and turkey)

skull

replicas of human and animal teeth

real human and animal teeth

shoes with Velcro straps

shoes to tie

boots to lace

buttons to sort

bathtub or shower faucets

hair cuttings from a stylist or barber

vegetables rooting in water

soap shapes to sort by shape, texture,
    color, and scent

bath toys to sort by size

Outdoors

helmets

work gloves

hard hats

binoculars

periscopes

telescopes

musical instruments

balls of many sizes

beanbags to toss

riding vehicles

disposable moist towelettes

tricycles

rhythm band instruments

herb and flower garden

megaphones

wind chimes

Technology

microscopes

stereo speakers to take apart

software or website that shows
  body parts

audio devices with headphones

rain sticks

Sand, Water, and Construction

water hose and sprinkler

wading pool

water for cleaning toys

sandpaper for sanding rough blocks
  of wood

birdbath

buckets of soapy water and sponges
  for washing

objects that sink and float

eyedroppers and colorful water

ice to observe melting

spray bottles of water

The Parts of Me!

LEARNING OBJECTIVES

- Children will identify visible body parts by their correct names.

- Children will show respect for differences in individual appearance.

- Children will practice behavior that protects their bodies (for example, using safety gear and wearing appropriate clothing).

Young children have a natural curiosity about their bodies, especially the external body parts that are visible. The concept of internal body parts is more difficult for preschoolers to understand. To introduce this concept, invite children to look at their faces and lips in a nonbreakable mirror. Ask them to open their mouths so they can see their tongues and teeth. Encourage children with visual impairments to feel their tongues and teeth with their fingers.

Introduce specific body parts one at a time, building on children's learning and experiences. For example, most children have experienced a cut or scraped knee, so they can understand that blood is inside of their bodies. Later they can explore the concept of a heart pumping blood throughout the body through blood vessels. Likewise, you can introduce the concept of bones creating a framework for the body.

Use correct terminology for body parts through the day. Hand-washing terms include *hands, fingers, skin, fingernails,* and *wrists.* Songs like the "Hokey Pokey" and games like Simon Says offer opportunities for children to move while identifying *arms, legs, feet, elbows, toes,* and other body parts.

Young children may think pain is normal, and they may not cry even when seriously injured. By learning about and being able to identify body parts, children can more easily alert adults if they are hurt or injured. When a child says, "I don't feel good," knowing whether his head, stomach, or extremities (arms and legs) hurt is helpful. Watch for changes in behavior or actions, and encourage children to tell an adult when they are hurting. Model appropriate terminology; when a child falls, say, "You scraped your knee," rather than, "You have a boo-boo."

Being able to identify body parts also helps children understand and accept differences. Children can recognize differences in height, weight, skin color, hair color, and use of glasses or hearing aids. Although young children can see physical differences, they may need help understanding how they are alike and different.

Protecting one's body is another component of this topic. Help young children learn how to exercise and nurture their bodies while also protecting themselves. Introduce children to the idea that clothing helps us stay healthy. Warm clothing protects us from cold weather and wind, raincoats shield us from rain, lightweight clothing keeps us from getting too warm, long sleeves and pants protect us from sunrays, and shoes protect our feet and toes. Shoes also protect our feet from glass and other debris and from insect stings and bites.

Children have temperature preferences. Some children are comfortable in short sleeves year-round, while others want to wear sweaters year-round. Encourage children to recognize and express when they are uncomfortable (for example, feeling too hot or cold) and to take appropriate actions (such as taking off or putting on a jacket).

Children have limited control over what clothing is available to them. Encourage families to dress children in clothing that allows freedom of movement and in footwear that provides support for running and jumping. Some families may not have appropriate outerwear or clothing in appropriate sizes, but a child without a warm coat at school may simply be stating her preference. If a family is in need of clothing, you may want to check available program or community resources. When offering assistance to families, be sensitive to their feelings.

Be aware that clothing choices may be informed by children's family, cultural, or religious backgrounds. Clothing is a significant part of individual and group identification. Learn the correct terminology for and significance of special clothing used by families in your classroom and community. As long as children's safety and health are not at risk, accept family choices for clothing.

VOCABULARY

ankle	eyes	neck	stomach
armpit	forehead	nose	thigh
calf	head	nostril	tongue
cheek	heel	palm	wrist
chest	hip	shin	
earlobe	knee	shoulder	
elbow	lips	skin	

CREATING THE ENVIRONMENT

■ Encourage self-help skills, independence, and decision making by providing each child with an accessible place to hang or store coats, hats, and other clothing.

■ Have extra clothing (such as jackets, hats, and closed shoes) available for children who do not come to class with appropriate clothing for outdoor play.

■ Include a wide variety of clothes and accessories for dramatic play so children become familiar with clothing for different activities and celebrations and clothing from different cultures.

■ Provide nonbreakable mirrors in hand-washing areas to encourage children to focus on their own hygiene.

■ Make sure child-size helmets are available to children every time they use a wheeled toy. Kneepads and elbow pads, along with helmets, offer protection when children go ice-skating or in-line skating and when they use riding toys or scooters.

■ Provide protective gear as needed for various activities. Gloves are great for picking up trash or digging in the sand. Safety goggles offer protection during woodworking activities.

■ Encourage sun safety every day, all year long. Sunglasses and wide-brimmed hats help prevent damage from sunrays. Long sleeves and pants can provide sun protection while still being comfortable and cool.

EVALUATION

■ Do children increasingly use correct names for body parts?

■ Can children compare their height, skin color, and hair color to other people's?

■ Do children use protective clothing and safety gear, such as helmets and kneepads or sunglasses and hats?

■ Do children use language and actions to show acceptance of their bodies and the bodies of others?

■ Do children ask for or initiate dressing appropriately for weather and outside play?

CHILDREN'S ACTIVITIES

Tickle My Toes

Play the song "Tickle My Toes" by Justin Roberts. Ask children if they know what *tickle* means. Listen to their tickle stories, commenting now and then. Tell them that when someone is touched softly or tickled, the person may want to move away, but sometimes tickling may cause the person to smile or laugh. Using a craft feather, softly tickle your own wrist. Ask children if they want you to tickle their wrists, and then tickle any volunteers with the feather. Ask them how it feels. Let children know that you are going to give each of them a feather. After passing out the feathers, ask them to tickle their own visible body parts, one at a time, as you name them. Start with the body parts children are most likely to know, such as finger, toe, face, ear, nose, mouth, arm, leg, foot, stomach, knee, and elbow. Then add body parts they are less likely to know, such as wrist, ankle, shin, chest, palm, hip, back, eyebrow, thigh, shoulder, neck, chin, earlobe, and armpit. If they do not know a body part, tickle yours to show them. Play the game again, adding new body parts each time. To add a math element, count the feathers as you distribute and collect them.

💬 ➕ 🏃 ❤️

❗ Safety Note: Let children know to keep their feathers away from their eyes when tickling their faces and to tickle only the outside of their ears, noses, and mouths.

MATERIALS
- a recording of "Tickle My Toes" by Justin Roberts, an audio device for playing music, and one craft feather per child

OTHER IDEAS
- Play traditional games like Simon Says and sing traditional songs like "Head, Shoulders, Knees, and Toes" and the "Hokey Pokey" so children can practice recognizing body parts.
  🎼 💬 🏃 ❤️

- Help children use their body parts to make sounds, such as clapping, snapping, humming, and flapping. Challenge them to come up with sounds by asking questions like, "What sounds can your feet make?"
  🎼 💬 🏃 ❤️

- Play the song "Smart Parts" by Justin Roberts, and then ask children which body parts they think are their smart parts.
  🎼 💬 🏃

- Read and discuss *Me and My Amazing Body* by Joan Sweeney.
  💬 🧪

The Body as a Work of Art

Arrange a trip to see various art representations of bodies. Prepare children to look at the many ways bodies are represented and displayed. Ask open-ended questions to encourage observation and discussion. Encourage children to compare the various representations in terms of size, materials, realness, and so on. Let children sketch or take pictures of what they see. Consider the following locations for visits: an art shop or museum with sculptures, photographs, drawings, and paintings; an art class with works in progress; a lawn and garden store with statues, water fountains, and plaques; a clothing store with mannequins; a doll store; a gift store with figurines; a dance studio or recital hall; a garden to see scarecrows; and a public park with monuments or statues.

MATERIALS
- paper, pencils, and a camera

OTHER IDEAS

- Give a doll to each child. Ask children how the dolls' body parts are like their own body parts. Ask how the dolls' body parts are different from their own body parts.

- Give a stuffed animal to each child. Ask children how the stuffed animals' body parts are like their own body parts. Ask how the stuffed animals' body parts are different from their own body parts. Then ask children to compare their fingers to the fingers of another child. Let children compare other visible body parts with one another, and encourage them to be accepting of differences.

- Play "Just an Old Jalopy" by the Cat's Pajamas. Visit a car garage or auto-body shop, and talk about the various car bodies and parts. Ask an employee to tell children the names of a car's body parts and to show them the tools used to keep the car's parts running smoothly.

- Visit a museum, medical facility, or other location to see skeletons and bones. Talk briefly about the parts of the body they cannot see.

Making Bodies

For this activity, plan to work with one small group of children at a time. Tell each small group of children that they are going to make a body and can draw or paint it on paper, mold it out of modeling clay, or create it with stuffing and dress-up clothes (like a scarecrow). Encourage them to decide what kind of body they want to make and ask whether they want to make the body alone or together. Help them identify the materials they need, and help them make a plan. Facilitate and support children as needed. Play the song "Skin" by Angie Bolton and Dennis Westphall. Talk with children about the importance of skin on the bodies they are making, and encourage them to include as many body parts as possible.

■ materials identified by children, a recording of "Skin" by Angie Bolton and Dennis Westphall, and an audio device for playing music

OTHER IDEAS

■ Invite a medical professional to visit the classroom with charts, X-rays, and models of the human body.

■ Invite a veterinarian to visit the classroom with animal pictures, charts, X-rays, and models of animal bodies.

■ Read *Contemplating Your Bellybutton* by Jun Nanao.

■ Help children cut out linked paper dolls. Provide paper strips, and show children how to fold the strip back and forth into four equal parts. With the paper folded, help children draw a picture of a child with arms outstretched, touching the sides of the paper. Provide a template for them to draw around if needed. Have children cut around the outline, except where the arms touch the edges.

Protection

Play the song "Driving in My Car" by the Cat's Pajamas. Tell children that the outsides of their bodies protect the insides of their bodies by keeping out germs and holding their bodies together. Explain that our outside parts (such as our eyes and skin) sometimes need protecting and that protecting our outside parts helps us stay healthy. Show items used to protect the body, and allow children to try on some of the items to demonstrate how they are used. Invite them to share what they know about the items. Ask additional questions, such as "Have you ever worn one of these?" and "Who might wear this?" and "Why might someone wear this?" Explain that we need to protect our bodies from harm. Add materials to interest areas for follow-up role playing and for actual use in activities such as riding trikes or woodworking.

MATERIALS

- a recording of "Driving in My Car" by the Cat's Pajamas, an audio device for playing music, and a collection of safety items (such as goggles, sunglasses, helmets, kneepads, elbow pads, mouth guards, steel-toe shoes, rain boots, sunscreen, sun hats, insect repellent, dust masks, long pants, back supports, swimming earplugs, winter coats, umbrellas, adhesive bandages, safety vests, life jackets, rubber gloves, shower safety grips, and so on)

OTHER IDEAS

- Have children sort baskets of clothing according to weather conditions, such as rainy, sunny and hot, and snowy. Ask children to explain their decisions. Remember that children experience temperatures differently from one another, just as adults do.

- Set up a safety gear store in the classroom as a special interest area. Involve children in designing the space and deciding what items to include, how much each item should cost, and in writing the job description for the store clerks.

- Visit a workplace where employees wear protective equipment or clothing, or invite a worker to visit the classroom wearing protective gear for children to see and ask questions about.

- Visit a store that sells protective materials and check out the variety and prices, or ask a store manager to bring a sampling of safety gear to the classroom to show children what each item is used for and tell them what it costs.

Unpacking

Select suitcases of various sizes, shapes, and materials with varying handles and designs. Pack each one with clean clothes for dolls, children, and adults that are used for work, play, and dress-up. Include clothes for all seasons and from many cultures. Talk with children about how the suitcases are alike and different. Let them move the suitcases around and check to see how heavy they are. Point out that just as the suitcases are different from one another, so are people. See if they can name some of the ways they are different from one another. If needed, ask questions like, "Is everyone's hair the same color?" and "Do the clothes everyone is wearing look the same?" Involve children in opening the suitcases and removing clothes one garment at a time. Ask children to describe the clothes. Talk about the size body that might have worn the clothes and in what kind of weather. After each item is discussed, have a child put the garment in a clothes hamper. Leave some clothes and empty suitcases in a designated place for children to use in role playing.

💬 ➕ ❤️

MATERIALS

- a variety of suitcases, a wide variety of clothing (including clothes for various types of weather and various sizes of people), and clothes hampers

OTHER IDEAS

- Read and discuss *People* by Peter Spier. Help children understand that we all have unique body types and that we should be respectful of differences.

  ➕ ⚗️ ❤️

- Add to the environment a variety of representations of the human body, such as paper dolls, wooden dolls, doll babies, fashion dolls, action figures, photos of people, and figurines. Ask each child to find a "body" in the classroom and bring it back to the group. Encourage children to compare the bodies they collected and to identify the ways they are alike and different from one another.

  💬 ⚗️ ❤️

- Help children sort themselves according to body similarities and differences. Assist them in seeing that they may have hair color in common with one child and height in common with another. Have children help you count the number of children according to hair color, height, skin color, shoe size, and other features so the information can be put on a chart.

  💬 ➕ ❤️

■ Distribute a storybook to each child. Ask children to look at the characters in the story to see what their body parts look like. Encourage them to compare the physical attributes of characters in one book to the physical attributes of characters in another (such as in hair color, hair length, height, weight, age, skin color, and so on).

Body Buddies

Meet with children in small groups. Explain that they are to come up with a way to show other children in the class what they have learned about bodies. They can create and sing a song, make a book and show it, draw a picture and tell about it, present a puppet show, or use any other ideas they have. Assure them that you will provide materials and help them. Support each group, asking questions to help children focus on the content about body parts, protecting their bodies, and accepting differences in others. Arrange a time for each group to share their experiences. Film the activity so children can watch themselves, and make the recording available to their families.

MATERIALS

■ materials identified by children, a video camera, and a viewing device for the video

OTHER IDEAS

■ Invite another class or family members to see the creations children have made to demonstrate their understanding of body parts.

■ Let children use a computer or an application on a multi-touch mobile device to write and illustrate a book about body parts.

■ Ask children, one at a time, to play "school" with you. Let them know you want to be the student and that you want them to teach you about body parts. As you play, evaluate what each child knows.

■ Place pictures of body parts in a box. Ask each child to take a picture out of the box and then share what the body part is and how to take care of it.

FAMILY INFORMATION

THE PARTS OF ME!

Young children are curious about their bodies and enjoy naming and counting their body parts. Movement games, such as Simon Says and Follow the Leader, and movement songs, such as the "Hokey Pokey," are fun ways to join children in movement as they learn the names of body parts.

Help your child use correct terms rather than nicknames for body parts. This skill is very important for times when your child is injured or does not feel well. Knowing the correct terms will help your child tell you, a teacher, or a doctor what part of her or his body is hurting.

PROTECT YOUR BODY

Clothing helps protect our bodies. Dress your child in layers of clothing that can be removed if he or she gets hot while playing. Choose shoes that cover the entire foot and that close with ties or self-stick straps. Shoes that support and protect feet allow your child to run faster, jump higher, and have more fun!

Teach your child how to protect body parts. Helmets help prevent head and facial injuries and are worn while bicycling, skating, or skateboarding. Elbow, knee, and wrist pads can prevent serious joint and bone injuries. Many sports and athletic activities also require protective gear.

Many communities have bike safety events and may provide free helmets. Check with your local police or fire department or city hall office.

Remember that your child watches what you do. Modeling safe behavior is the best way to teach young children!

FAMILY ACTIVITY

Ask your child to name the body parts shown in the pictures on the left. Then help your child draw a line from each body part on the left to the item on the right that protects or goes with that body part.

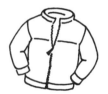

My Five Senses!

LEARNING OBJECTIVES

- Children will identify ways they use their senses.
- Children will practice behavior that protects their sight and hearing.
- Children will show respect for people who do not have full use of all senses.

An exploration of the five senses can introduce children to the way body parts work. Children recognize external body parts (such as eyes, ears, noses, tongues, and fingers), and through hands-on activities, they can associate those parts with specific functions. Children learn by using their senses and exploring how body parts work together; for example, serving crisp cereal with milk allows children to see the food, feel the difference between touching dry cereal and then wet milk, hear the cereal crackle as milk is added, and smell and taste the cereal with and without milk.

Some children may not have full use of all their senses, or they may not have yet developed an awareness of their senses. Other children may rely heavily on certain senses while ignoring others. Sensitivity may also change due to illnesses or external conditions; for example, when children or adults have colds, their senses of hearing, smell, and taste may change.

We use our senses daily. We use vision, smell, and taste when we eat. We rely on vision and hearing when crossing a street, and we use touch and vision when working a puzzle. Provide activities and opportunities that encourage children to use and learn through all their senses. In this manner, children with different sensitivities and abilities can participate and contribute to the classroom experience.

Help children understand the use and importance of the five senses, and help them learn ways to protect the parts of their bodies connected to the senses. Help children learn to protect their hearing by limiting the volume of music, especially when in a closed area (such as a vehicle) or when using headphones. Help them learn to protect their vision by wearing goggles and sunglasses when appropriate and by not looking directly at the sun or bright lights.

VOCABULARY

binoculars	goggles	periscope	taste
Braille	hearing	scent	telescope
earplug	hearing aid	sense	texture
feel	magnifier	sight	vision
flavor	megaphone	smell	
fragrance	microscope	sound	
glasses	odor	sunglasses	

CREATING THE ENVIRONMENT

- Provide a variety of objects for children to explore using their five senses, such as texture boards, scratch-and-sniff samples, musical instruments, and colorful puzzles.

- In the outdoor play area, include wind chimes, various surfaces for play (such as grass, sand, and concrete), and live nontoxic and fragrant plants. Designate a garden area for edible plants.

- Have protective gear, including safety goggles (for use during woodworking activities) and sunglasses, accessible to children.

- Make headphones accessible to children to encourage listening. Monitor their use of headphones; teach children to keep the volume low.

EVALUATION

- Can children discuss their body parts and associate them with their senses?

- Do children show curiosity and interest in using their senses?

- Do children protect their hearing by adjusting volume controls appropriately?

- Do children protect their sight by wearing goggles or sunglasses in appropriate situations?

- Do children show sensitivity to people with limited use of their senses?

CHILDREN'S ACTIVITIES

Animal Kingdom

Give children toy animals, and ask them to show you the animals' eyes, ears, noses, mouths, tongues, hands, and feet (or paws, hooves, and so on). Engage them in a discussion about how the animals might use these parts of their bodies. Then ask children to describe how they use their own eyes, ears, noses, mouths, feet, and hands. Introduce the term *senses,* and explain that we use our senses to learn, work, and play.

❗ Safety Note: Check all toy animals to ensure they do not have loose parts that children can dislodge, insert into their mouths, and choke on. All toys should be cleaned and sanitized regularly.

MATERIALS
- one toy animal (stuffed, plastic, or wooden) per child

OTHER IDEAS
- Read and discuss a book with animal characters. Encourage children to share what they think the animals see, hear, smell, taste, and touch.

- Provide animal puppets, and let children demonstrate how each animal uses its senses.

- Give each child a doll. Have children identify the body parts associated with the senses, and then ask each child to make up a story about how his doll will use one of its senses.

- Read and discuss *My Five Senses* by Aliki. Encourage children to share how they feel about their senses.

Baking Bread

Let children assist in preparing bread for baking. After they have washed their hands, let them examine the bread maker. Show children the recipe, and let them feel the ingredients. Involve them in measuring and mixing. Ask them questions such as "How much bread do you think this will make?" and "How do you think the bread maker works?" Begin baking bread at a time that will allow children to hear the machine work, peek through its window, and smell the bread baking. If you have access to an oven, make bread again and let the children knead it before rising and baking. After a taste test of the baked bread, discuss the taste. Provide a variety of toppings, including flavored butters, honey, and jellies. Make additional loaves so children can again feel the ingredients, hear the sounds, see the sights, smell the bread baking, and taste the final product.

MATERIALS

- a bread maker, an illustrated recipe card, ingredients to make bread, measuring cups, measuring spoons, a knife, serving plates, napkins, and toppings

OTHER IDEAS

- Provide a sample of foods that taste sour, sweet, salty, and bitter for a tasting party. Encourage children to describe the tastes and to share which ones they like and do not like. Create a class chart indicating children's preferences.

- Visit flower shops or nurseries so children can smell flowers, describe their fragrances, and discuss favorites. Alternately, bring fragrant flowers to the classroom for smelling. Tell children that some smells are pleasant and some are not. See if they can name some things that stink.

- Grow an herb garden so children can taste and smell a variety of herbs. Discuss the experience.

- Read *The Holes in Your Nose* by Genichiro Yagyu, and talk about ways to take care of noses (for example, by wearing a dust mask, blowing properly with both nostrils open, and never putting anything into the nose).

Satin Sheets

Provide an air mattress and several sheets made from a variety of materials. Making the sheets visually attractive adds another element for the senses. Large pieces of cloth also can be used with or without the air mattress. Change the sheets every day for at least a week, and encourage children to feel the "sheet of the day" with many of their body parts. Prompt them to discuss how the sheets feel on their fingers, toes, elbows, and knees. Explain that the sheets are made of different materials and that some people like one material better than another.

MATERIALS

- an air mattress and textured sheets or cloths made of various materials (such as satin, silk, rayon, polyester, flannel, cotton, jersey, netting, burlap, corduroy, and fur)

OTHER IDEAS

- Fill containers with objects and liquids that provide stimulating— and safe—tactile experiences. Allow children to explore the containers' contents and to describe what they feel. Help them recognize that they may like the way some things feel but not like the way other things feel.

- Fill a large box with fabric pieces of various textures, and encourage children to get into the box to feel the fabrics. See how many pieces of fabric children can count. The strips of fabric can be recycled to the art interest area when children tire of the sensory box.

- Let children use their feet to feel. Start by having children step in a plastic dishpan (or other container) filled with plain water. Vary the experience by changing the water temperature and depth or by adding supplements such as bubble bath or bath oil. A water foot massager can extend the tactile experience with bubbles.

- Read *Feel the Wind* by Arthur Dorros. Help children recognize the wind by turning on a fan (without exposed blades) so they can feel blowing air. Discuss the story, and explore the idea that wind can cool us down, help dry clothes, spread seeds, and even generate energy (windmills). Point out that windy weather can sometimes be unpleasant, frightening, or even dangerous. Allow time to hear their reactions.

Art Appreciation

Collect diverse pieces of art that look and feel different from one another. Place the art throughout the classroom, in the hall, in bathrooms, and outside. Place an envelope beside each piece of artwork. On the front of each envelope, write the corresponding artist's name and the title of the work. If the artist isn't credited on the piece, write "Unknown" for the artist's name. If a work is not named, write "Untitled" or let the children choose a name.

Discuss the characteristics of the art with children, and ask them questions about how each piece looks and feels. Tell children about each artist. Ask children to vote for their favorite pieces of artwork by placing strips of paper with their names on them in the appropriate envelopes. Assist children as needed with writing their names on strips of paper. Let children help count the names in the envelopes to see which piece of artwork received the most votes. Stress that it is acceptable for each of them to like different artwork.

MATERIALS

- a variety of artwork (including paintings, drawings, photographs, cards, posters, statues, sculptures, figurines, mobiles, pottery, garden bells, pinwheels, children's artwork, embroidery, calendar and magazine pictures, wood carvings, stained glass, wall hangings, rugs, quilts, beadwork, books of artwork, and jewelry), envelopes, pencils, and paper

OTHER IDEAS

- Provide tools that enhance sight (such as binoculars, magnifiers, microscopes, and telescopes). Encourage children to learn about each tool and to use the tools to look at the art collection, watch birds, and explore nature outside.

- Play the song "Get Me Some Glasses" by Justin Roberts, and listen to the words. Explain how some people need glasses to see well (far away or up close), but others do not.

- Read and discuss *Norman the Doorman* by Don Freeman.

- Provide a simple woodworking activity, such as sanding wood for an art project. Require children to wear goggles to protect their eyes. Discuss with children the importance of taking care of their eyes by wearing goggles, wearing sunglasses outside, and never looking directly into the sun or bright lights.

A Little Louder Now

Invite children to dance while you play "Shout" by the Isley Brothers. After the song, tell children in a loud but pleasant voice that some sounds are loud. Tell them that some sounds are too loud and can hurt their ears. Slowly lowering your voice with each word, say that some sounds are soft. Ask children to name loud and soft sounds. Tell children to watch and listen as you clap your hands. Sit and clap very softly. Partially stand up and clap a little louder. Then stand up all the way and clap very loudly. Invite children to clap with you. Next, teach children to watch your hand and to clap softly when it is low and to clap louder as it gets higher. Try moving from very soft to very loud both gradually and quickly. As a follow-up, use this technique for singing, chanting rhymes, stomping, and playing instruments.

MATERIALS
- a recording of "Shout" by the Isley Brothers and an audio device for music

OTHER IDEAS

- Play a sample of music from different genres (such as classical, folk, blues, jazz, reggae, and so on), and ask children to indicate whether they like each one by giving a thumbs up or a thumbs down. With the children, count the number of thumbs up and thumbs down for each selection, and record the number on a chart to review with them after listening to each selection.

- Provide tools that enhance sound, such as stethoscopes, children's microphones, tin cans with connecting string, and funnels. Encourage children to explore the tools and to discuss their results.

- Show children examples of ear- and hearing-protection devices (such as swimming earplugs for keeping out water, winter earmuffs for keeping out cold, and earplugs and earmuffs for working in loud environments). Explain that loud sounds can damage the ears, whether the sounds are heard outside, inside, or through headphones.

- Show children headphones and an audio device for playing music. Play music or a story without the head-phones, and let children watch you increase and decrease the volume; help them decide what is too low and what is too loud. Use a sticker, colored tape, or paint to show the acceptable volume range, and allow children to practice adjusting the volume when listening with head-phones.

Helpful Tools

Arrange for a guide or hearing service dog to visit the classroom so children can watch the dog work and learn what service dogs do for people. Prepare children in advance by letting them know the dog will be working and that it is not a pet. To arrange a visit, check with individuals who have a guide or hearing dog, a program specializing in training service dogs, or families who foster puppies until they are old enough to enter the specialized training. As an alternative, show photos or videos of service dogs, and tell children that the dogs are working to help people who cannot see or hear. Give a few examples of ways service dogs help people, such as by stopping at a curb so a person who is blind does not fall, guiding a person who is blind away from low-hanging trees or other obstacles they cannot see, and letting a person who is deaf know if the phone or doorbell is ringing or if someone is calling her name. Ask children what they think about service dogs.

MATERIALS

- photographs or videos of guide and hearing service dogs and a viewing device for the videos

OTHER IDEAS

- Ask children how they use their ears. Prompt them with questions until they mention things like hearing music, stories, traffic, dogs barking, and other people talking. Ask children to participate in an experiment to understand a little bit about what it is like to be unable to hear well. Provide earplugs or earmuffs, or have children cover their ears, as you whisper a set of directions for them to follow. You might ask them to jump up and down four times, turn around slowly, and clap their hands six times. Explain how people who are deaf or hearing impaired can do many things well, but they may need tools to help them (see below for a list of tools).

- Ask children how they use their eyes. Prompt them with questions until they mention things like seeing where to walk, finding toys, seeing friends, and so on. Ask children to participate in an experiment to understand a little bit about what it is like to be unable to see well. Provide eye masks or darkened glasses, or have children hold their hands over their eyes. Be sensitive to children who are fearful of covering their eyes. Give children a set of simple directions to follow while their eyes are covered. You might ask them to take three small steps forward, turn around, sit down, and shake hands with a friend. Explain how people who are visually impaired can do many things, but they may need tools to help them (see below for a list of tools).

- Show children a variety of tools used by the visually impaired, such as a pair of glasses, a book in Braille, a cane, and a talking watch. Initiate a conversation about the tools. If possible, invite a guest who is visually impaired to show the tools and talk about how they help him perform tasks.

- Show children a variety of tools used by the hearing impaired, such as a hearing aid, an amplified phone, and flashing alerts. If possible, invite someone to teach the children a few words in sign language, or use a children's book (such as the Sign and Sing Along books by Annie Kubler) to show the signs. Talk about the ways sign language and other tools can be helpful to individuals with hearing impairments.

FAMILY INFORMATION

MY FIVE SENSES!

Children learn by using their five senses—sight, hearing, smell, taste, and touch. They taste and smell new foods. When learning a new skill, they hear your directions and see you demonstrate the activity. Children learn through touch that items can be warm or cold. As you talk about the five senses, children also learn about body parts: eyes, ears, nose, tongue, and fingers.

One way to teach your child how senses work together is by cooking a favorite food. Ask your child questions, such as "Do you smell the cookies?" and "Do they look like they are done?" and "They feel warm but not too hot; should we taste one?"

THE FIVE SENSES AND SAFETY

The five senses are important to your child's safety. Teach your child to stop, look, and listen before crossing streets. Remember that children under the age of six still need your help in crossing a street.

The senses are also used for fire safety. You might tell your child, "If there is a fire, you may hear the alarm. You may smell the smoke. Get out of the house! Feel the door before you open it. If the door is warm or hot, get out through a window or another door."

PROTECT EYES AND EARS

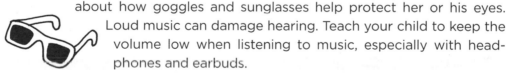

Children can learn ways to protect their sight and hearing. Talk to your child about how goggles and sunglasses help protect her or his eyes. Loud music can damage hearing. Teach your child to keep the volume low when listening to music, especially with headphones and earbuds.

FAMILY ACTIVITY

Encourage your child to color the pictures below, and then discuss the items in each picture and whether you can taste, touch, hear, smell, or see each one.

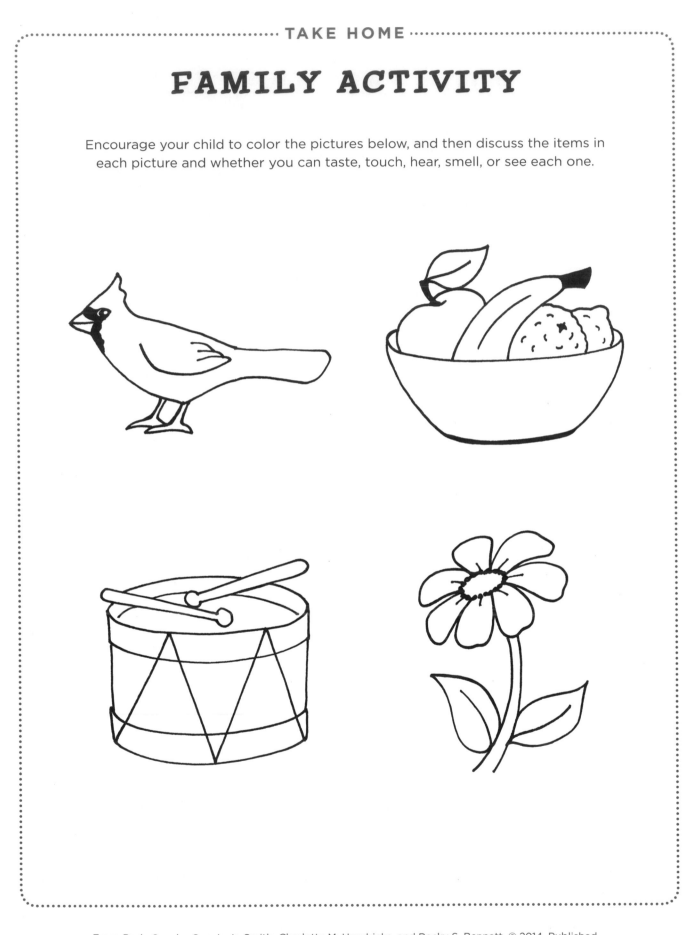

Keeping All My Body Parts Clean!

- Children will communicate ways to clean their bodies.

- Children will show acceptance of differences in hair (such as in texture, color, and style).

- Children will communicate that cleanliness (for example, of body, hair, and clothes) helps prevent diseases (for example, by removing germs and keeping them well).

Cleanliness is important for preventing infections in cuts and scratches, irritated skin, and sores. Proper hygiene practices (for example, bathing) are important for protecting us from communicable diseases. Bacteria, viruses, or parasites can cause skin conditions, such as impetigo, ringworm, and scabies; and the transmission of these conditions is increased by poor hygiene. Cleanliness can also promote self-esteem in children.

Many young children have little regard for their personal appearance. They may not care whether they have brushed their teeth or combed their hair, and they may prefer a dirty favorite shirt over a clean one. Nearly all children will occasionally arrive to class looking a little messy or untidy. This is normal and no cause for concern.

Some children, however, may wear the same clothes several days in a row, and the condition of the clothes may suggest they have not been washed overnight. Some children also may have an odor that comes from their bodies or their unwashed clothes.

The reasons why families may have inadequate or inappropriate hygiene practices are diverse. Some families do not have easy access to running water or laundry facilities. Other families may not have funds to purchase soap, personal hygiene products, and laundry detergent and services. Poor hygiene can result from a lack of information or knowledge about the importance of cleanliness to children's health. And different cultures and families have different beliefs about hygiene; many families do not consider daily or even weekly bathing to be necessary.

Likewise, the idea of what constitutes appropriate hair grooming varies greatly. Hair grooming may involve combing or brushing, using a pick, or putting in barrettes and ribbons. Children with very short hair may just need to "brush" over their head with a dry cloth to remove sand or dirt. Be sensitive to the various hair-grooming techniques that are based on the characteristics of hair (such as straight or curly, oily or dry, and coarse or smooth). Hairstyles may also vary based on personal or cultural preferences. Use correct terminology for the classroom population's hairstyles, haircuts, hair care procedures, and hair products.

Clean, well-groomed hair is important for reasons other than appearance. Dry scalp (dandruff) can cause itching, and itching can cause skin conditions such as eczema and impetigo. Parasites such as head lice can also live in the hair; spotting and removing lice and nits (lice eggs) is easier in well-groomed hair. Head lice prefer clean, dry hair with a smooth texture so they can attach their nits to the hair shafts. Lice do not like hair with a coarse texture.

VOCABULARY

barber	detergent	length	soap
bath	dry	oily	straight
braid	faucet	pick	towel
brush	grooming	plumbing	wash
clean	hairstyle	salon	
comb	hygiene	shampoo	
curly	laundry	shower	

CREATING THE ENVIRONMENT

- Encourage children to groom their hair when it is appropriate. After playing outside, children may want to brush, comb, or shake sand and dirt from their hair. Have children use individual brushes, combs, and picks that can be stored in their individual storage spaces after use.

- Nonbreakable mirrors may encourage children to look at and care for their hair and to wash their faces when needed.

- Keep extra clean clothes in the classroom so they're available for children who need them. If necessary, assist children in putting on clean clothes and storing the dirty clothes for return.

EVALUATION

- Do children talk about the importance of bathing and hair care?
- During play, do children demonstrate bathing and hair care with dolls and toy people?
- Do children talk about hair differences in accepting ways?
- During pretend play, do children demonstrate care for clothing (for example, by doing laundry and changing clothes when dirty)?
- During pretend play, do children use props such as soap and empty bubble bath containers?

CHILDREN'S ACTIVITIES

Bathtub and Shower Model

Show children photographs of various styles of bathtubs and showers from supplier brochures and catalogs. Ask children why people take baths and showers, and reinforce answers that address getting clean, feeling good, smelling good, and staying healthy. Explain that getting dirty is all right when playing and working, but washing up afterward is important. Tell children you want them to think of ways they can make a pretend shower and bathtub that can be used in the classroom for playing. Encourage them to think of the materials they need and the steps involved in creating a shower or tub. Ask specific questions to help them create realistic and life-size models, such as "How will you know what size to make the bathtub?" Use a tape measure to help them measure the length and height needed. Keep notes of children's ideas on a large sheet of paper so you can refer to it as you guide them. Continue the activity when you are able to provide the materials requested (or adequate substitutes) and the guidance to help children succeed. Place the completed models in an appropriate place to encourage role playing. Take pictures or film a video of children as they work on and play with the models. Put the pictures or video where children and families can view them.

MATERIALS

- photographs of bathtubs and showers, materials children request and supplements you choose (such as large cardboard boxes, old plumbing fixtures, pipes, paint, glue, paint-color samples to use as tiles, a shower curtain, and a dowel rod or long stick for hanging the shower curtain), measuring tools, a large sheet of paper, a pen or marker, a camera or video camera, and a viewing device for the video (if needed)

OTHER IDEAS

- Visit a bathroom facility in the classroom building or on the grounds that includes a bathtub or shower. Let children operate the faucets to see how they work. Ask children questions to help them examine the details. Let children take pictures and measure the tub and shower.

- Assist children in creating a class recording of water sounds to listen to when they role-play bathing or relaxing. Use running water from sinks, water fountains, or other available water sources. Let children operate the recording device.

- Listen to the song "Crowded Tub" by Gilda Radner, and read *No More Water in the Tub!* by Tedd Arnold.

- Visit a locker room, and let children take a shower with their swimsuits on.

❗Safety Note: Be sure the locker room and shower floor have been cleaned and disinfected. Children should wear shoes appropriate for use in the shower.

Baby Bath

Show children a washable baby doll and bathing supplies. Ask them why bathing babies is important, and listen for answers about getting babies clean, making them smell good, and keeping them healthy; listen for answers about babies being too little to bathe themselves. Point out that babies need help with things they have not yet learned to do. Ask children if they know how to bathe themselves, and reinforce the idea that they are able to do many things to keep themselves clean and healthy. Using a doll and a baby bathtub or dishpan, show children how to bathe a baby. Talk about the water temperature, and let children feel it. Talk about the depth of the water, and let children measure it with a ruler. Discuss the amount of soap to use and how to lather, rinse, and dry each body part. Point out that the baby's ears need to be washed but that nothing smaller than a finger in a washcloth should be put into the baby's ears or their own. Provide bathing materials and dolls for children to use for role playing.

MATERIALS
- a washable baby doll, a baby bathtub or dishpan, clean water, soap, a washcloth, a towel, and a ruler

OTHER IDEAS

- Show a variety of bath toys (including color-changing bath tablets, bath crayons, squirt toys, and float toys) and accessories (including bubble bath, bar soap, bath beads, skin-exfoliating mitts, bath pillows, loofah back brushes, pumice stones, mesh bath sponges, a shower bench, a bath mat, and safety grips). Ask children what they know about each item, and briefly explain any item children are not familiar with.

- Encourage children to make a book they can share with younger children to help them understand how to take a bath. Encourage children to include all body parts. Assist with writing, and suggest illustrations to make the subject easy for younger children to understand. Arrange for children to read their book to younger children in the program.

- Play the song "Bathtime" by Raffi, and sing along with it.

- Read and discuss books on hygiene, such as *Big Smelly Bear* by Britta Teckentrup.

Washing Hair

Play the song "Henrietta's Hair" by Justin Roberts, and listen carefully to the words. Ask children if they think Henrietta needs her hair washed. Invite children to share what they know about washing hair. Encourage them to share how they feel about having their own hair washed, why people wash their hair, what supplies are needed to wash hair, and the steps in washing hair. After the discussion, show children the supplies for washing hair and a doll that needs a hair wash. Let children help fill up the baby bathtub or dishpan, one cup of warm water at a time. Invite one child to demonstrate how to wash the hair and keep the soap out of the doll's eyes. Then ask another child to demonstrate how to towel dry the hair. Ask a third child to show how to comb the hair. Encourage children to say soothing things to the doll so she remains calm. Make the doll and hair-washing supplies available so all the children can experience washing a doll's hair.

💬 🏃 ❤️

MATERIALS

- a recording of "Henrietta's Hair" by Justin Roberts, an audio device for music, a baby bathtub or dishpan, clean water, a cup for pouring water, baby shampoo, a towel, a comb, and a washable doll with hair

OTHER IDEAS

- Play the song "New Haircut" by Justin Roberts, and listen to the words. Visit a hairstylist or barber (licensed or in a school) to observe the work being done and the tools used. Draw children's attention to the hair washing and haircuts. Prior to the visit, help children come up with questions to ask the hairstylist or barber during the visit.

  💬 💻

- Go for a walk to look for hair on animals. Discuss with children the characteristics (such as short, long, or tangled) of the hair they see on animals, and ask what they think it would be like to wash that hair. Look for any cats that are washing themselves (or watch a video clip), and talk about how cats keep clean.

  🏃 ⚗️

- Visit a dog groomer or veterinarian, and observe a dog bath and nail clipping. Note all of the body parts that are washed and groomed, and discuss the tools used. Talk about the importance of cutting our finger- and toenails and washing around them.

Alternately, invite a pet owner to wash his dog at school for the children to observe.

■ Set up a birdbath so children can observe birds washing their feathers. Compare the birds to people taking a bath and washing their hair.

Hairstyles

Show children several dolls, including both males and females with different kinds of hair. Ask them how the dolls are alike and how they are different. If no one mentions the hair, ask specific questions, such as "How is this doll's hair different from this one's?" and "Which doll's hair is curly?" and "Which doll's hair do you like the best?" Help children see differences in the color, length, texture, and style of hair. Let children know that even though people may like one hair color or hairstyle better than another, we should treat everyone fairly regardless of their hair color or hairstyle.

💬 ➕ ❤️

MATERIALS
- dolls with different kinds of hair

OTHER IDEAS

- Encourage children to look in a non-breakable mirror and study and talk about their own hair. Ask questions about color, length, texture, style, and so on to prompt them to describe their hair.

  💬 ➕ ❤️

- Visit a store that sells dolls, or invite a doll collector to the classroom to show children a variety of doll hairstyles. Include male and female dolls. Prepare children for limited touching of some dolls, stressing that they should use their eyes instead of their hands.

  💬 ⚗️

- Visit a wig store, and look at the wide selection of wigs. Ask the clerk to explain to children how wigs are made and how to take care of them.

  💬 ⚗️ 💻

- Show children hair cuttings obtained from a hairstylist. Ask them if they know what you are holding. Let the children examine the hair under a microscope, with a magnifying glass, and with their naked eyes.

  💬 ⚗️ 💻

Hair Snapshots

Invite several guests to attend a hairstyle photo shoot and interview session in the classroom. Prepare a diverse guest list that includes males and females, both young people and old, and individuals of different ethnicities. Plan to have many colors, lengths, textures, and styles of hair represented. Invite a woman with short hair and a man with long hair. Include family members of children in the class. As guests are invited, prepare them for children's questions, such as "How do you take care of your hair?" and "Can I touch your hair?" Let children practice using a camera before the photo shoot. Show them photographs as examples of images that focus on hair. During the shoot, you and the children should take pictures of each guest for follow-up classroom discussions and activities. Photographs can show the front, side, and back views of the hair. Invite a local television or newspaper reporter to cover the event. Remember to obtain parent permission to include children's images or names in the media, including social media, such as Facebook.

MATERIALS
- a camera, photographs of hair taken in the classroom or from magazines

OTHER IDEAS

- Give children the opportunity to select and use materials (such as yarn and clay) to create a model of hair. Set up a viewing area for children to see one another's work.

- Let children make a collage of hairstyles by cutting pictures from old magazines and catalogs and gluing them however they desire to fill a poster. Ask them open-ended questions about the pictures they select.

- Encourage children to look at their own baby pictures and to discuss how their hair has changed.

- Read books about hair, such as *Ella Kazoo Will Not Brush Her Hair* by Lee Fox.

Rinse It, Wring It, Hang It

Select a few pieces of clean, washable clothing with readable care tags, and put them in a clothes hamper. Gather a small group of children, and have each of them get something out of the hamper. Ask them where they put their dirty clothes at home. After telling them that most clothing has a care tag sewn or printed inside, ask them what they think is on the tag. Once children locate the tags, read each one to them. Provide supplies for washing clothes, and let each child wash a piece of clothing by hand and then rinse it, wring it, and hang it on an indoor or outdoor clothesline. Allow children to feel and smell the clothes at various stages. Tell them that getting dirty is all right when playing or working, but changing into clean clothes after we take a bath is important. Stress that clean clothes help us smell good and feel better.

MATERIALS

■ clean washable clothes, a clothes hamper, a washtub or dishpan, clean water, hypoallergenic detergent, fabric softener, stain remover, a clothesline, and clothespins

OTHER IDEAS

■ Provide supplies for washing, and invite the children to wash, wring, and hang doll clothes.

■ Invite an employee from a dry-cleaning business to visit the classroom and explain the tools used to clean clothes without getting them wet. Encourage the visitor to show photographs and tools to help the children understand.

■ Visit a coin-operated laundry or the program's laundry room, and use the machines to wash and dry the classroom dress-up clothes. Examine how the washer and dryer work.

■ Provide a variety of empty and clean detergent and fabric softener containers and lids. Let the children match lids to the correct container and practice putting lids on and taking them off. While they play the matching game, talk with them about the importance of clean clothes.

FAMILY INFORMATION

KEEPING ALL MY BODY PARTS CLEAN!

Being clean helps children stay healthy. Washing and bathing helps prevent infection in cuts and scratches, irritated skin, and sores. Bathing also helps stop the spread of ringworm, scabies, and other diseases.

Make bath time fun! Soap bubbles and lather, floating toys, and a little splashing can all help children explore and learn. Help your child wash every part of her or his body—even behind the ears! Help your child dress in clean clothes after bathing.

Take your child with you when you shop for bathing supplies. Let your child help select items he or she needs to take a bath or shower.

KEEP BATH TIME SAFE

Never leave your child under age six alone in the bathtub! Young children can drown in just a few inches of water.

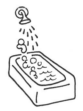

Children's skin is very tender; children can get a serious burn in just a few seconds. The temperature of hot water should be no more than 120 degrees Fahrenheit (49 degrees Celsius) when it comes out of the tap. You can control the water temperature by adjusting the water heater or by installing a temperature regulator.

HAIR CARE

Even young children can learn about hair care. Explain to your child how you care for your own hair and how you care for her or his hair. If your child is interested, let her or him participate in hair care, including washing, combing or picking, and adding products or accessories (such as gel, barrettes, or ribbons).

FAMILY ACTIVITY

Circle the pictures that go together in each row, or circle the one picture that doesn't belong with the others in the row. While assisting your child with this activity, discuss cleanliness and the activities and items that help us stay clean and healthy.

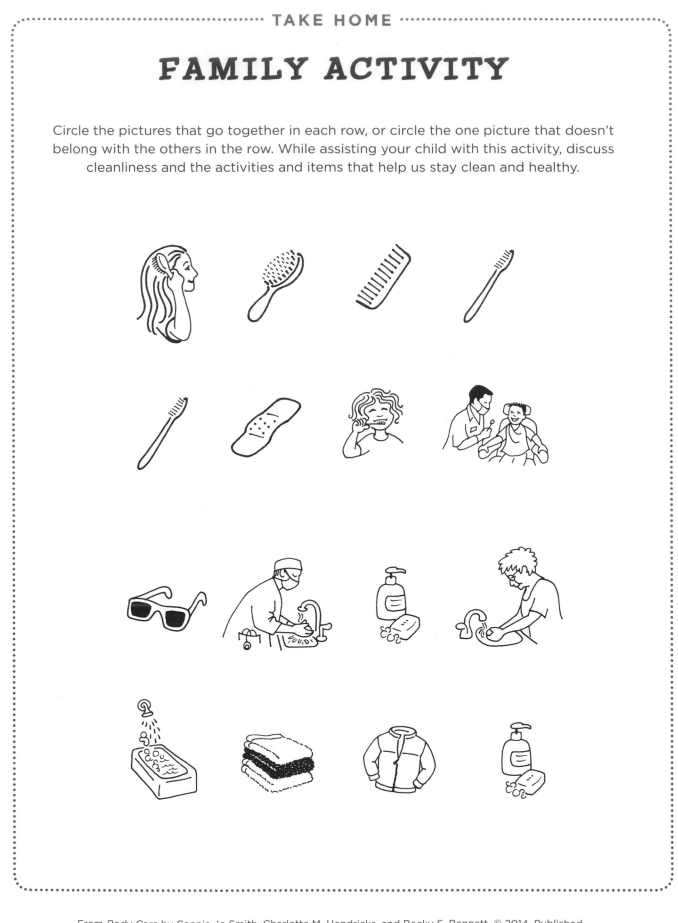

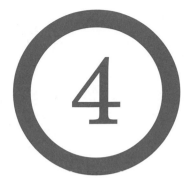

Taking Care of My Smile!

LEARNING OBJECTIVES

■ Children will practice toothbrushing, including using the correct technique and brushing at appropriate times.

■ Children will communicate why teeth are important (for example, for chewing, smiling, and talking).

■ Children will show or talk about how a dentist helps take care of their teeth.

Toothbrushing and flossing remove food from teeth. When food is not removed, bacteria grow and form plaque (a film on the teeth). The germs in plaque make acid; and when plaque clings to teeth, the acid can eat away at the outermost layer (the enamel) of the tooth, which can lead to decay (cavities).

Children (and adults) should brush their teeth thoroughly at least twice each day—after breakfast and before bedtime. Encourage children to brush their teeth, and help them develop toothbrushing skills by providing an opportunity for them to brush their teeth each day. For some children, this daily practice may be the only opportunity they have for toothbrushing, so brushing thoroughly is important. Help children follow this toothbrushing procedure:

1. Put a tiny (pea-size) amount of fluoride toothpaste on the toothbrush and wet the toothbrush under running water or in a disposable cup with water in it.

2. Place the toothbrush at an angle against the gums.

3. Gently move the brush, using a circular motion. Brush the outside, inside, and top of each tooth. Brush for at least two minutes.

4. Brush the tongue.

5. Spit the toothpaste into the sink or into the disposable cup.

Supervise children as they brush, and assist them if necessary. Encourage children to check their teeth after brushing. Older children may also floss their teeth.

If brushing is not possible, provide disposable cups and encourage children to swish and spit with water after eating. This action helps remove food particles and reduce bacteria in the mouth.

Young children should not use mouthwash or rinses, for they often swallow the fluid, which may contain alcohol, fluoride, or other ingredients. In large amounts, these ingredients can be harmful to young children.

What and when you eat are important in dental health. Snacking or consuming sweetened beverages throughout the day allows food to remain on teeth for long periods. When food is in the mouth, bacteria can grow, creating plaque.

Some foods stick to teeth more than others. The sugar in hard or sticky candy stays on teeth longer than the sugar in cake or chocolate bars. Dried, processed fruit snacks appear to be healthful, but they contain high amounts of sugar, which sticks to the teeth. Children may eat these foods occasionally, but having food, including sweets, only at meals or designated snacktimes—rather than throughout the day—is best.

Sugar is not the only problem; diet and regular sodas, energy drinks, sour gummy candies, and even fruits such as apples and grapes contain high amounts of acid. This acid can weaken the enamel on teeth. Encourage children to drink water and rinse teeth immediately after meals and snacks.

Children should visit a dentist at least every six months, or more often if needed. Discuss with children how dentists and dental hygienists help us take care of our teeth. Discuss points such as how children should open their mouths at the dentist, how a dental mirror helps the dentist see their teeth, and what special ways the dental professional will brush their teeth. Most dental clinics have environments and activities to make visits fun for children; many communities have pediatric dental clinics. Invite a dentist or dental hygienist from your community to talk with children about toothbrushing and visiting a dental clinic.

PREVENTING DENTAL INJURIES

Children may injure their teeth if they fall when skateboarding, in-line skating, or bicycling. Insist that children wear helmets to prevent dental and head injuries. A helmet should fit a child's head snugly and cover the forehead. If a child falls, the helmet—not the forehead—will hit the ground first and hold the child's face and teeth away from the ground.

If a tooth is broken or knocked out, collect all pieces of the tooth. Place the tooth in a wet cloth or a container of water, milk, or the child's own saliva (spit).

If the child is older, he may be able to hold the tooth in his mouth until you reach the dentist. Take the child and the tooth to a dentist immediately. With immediate treatment, the dentist may be able to save the child's tooth.

VOCABULARY

bad breath	enamel	orthodontist	swish
brush	floss	outside	toothache
cavity	fluoride	plaque	top
chew	gums	root	X-ray
circular	hygienist	smile	
decay	in between	spit	
dentist	inside	sticky	

CREATING THE ENVIRONMENT

- The ideal environment includes a child-size sink with running water. If a sink is not available, have children use a cup of water for rinsing and spitting.
- Provide each child with a child-size toothbrush with soft bristles. Label each toothbrush and storage case or slot with the child's name.
- Store toothbrushes in a manner that allows them to air-dry and prevents cross-contamination. Place toothbrushes in a receptacle bristle-ends up; do not allow toothbrushes to touch one another. Use covered net or screen storage containers to prevent access by insects.
- Provide children with individual toothpaste tubes labeled with their names. Another option is to distribute toothpaste to each child on waxed-paper squares or craft sticks. A single tube of toothpaste should not touch children's toothbrushes.
- Provide disposable cups for rinsing after brushing, if desired.
- Hang a nonbreakable mirror on the wall in the toothbrushing area so children can check their teeth.

EVALUATION

- Do children increasingly use the correct technique when brushing their teeth?
- Have children asked for or initiated brushing their teeth at appropriate times?
- Can children make statements about why their teeth are important?
- Do children include dental care in their play?
- Can children communicate the ways a dentist helps care for their teeth?

CHILDREN'S ACTIVITIES

Gum It

Ask children what they think the inside of a baby's mouth looks like and what they think babies eat. Ask them how the inside of a baby's mouth is different from their own mouths, and prompt them with questions until someone mentions teeth. Then invite a parent and her baby to visit the classroom. Prepare children to be quiet and gentle so the baby does not become frightened. In advance of the visit, help children come up with questions to ask the parent about the baby's mouth, such as "How do you clean the baby's gums?" and "What food can the baby eat?" and "When will the baby first go to the dentist?" After the visit, talk with children about how their teeth help them eat more foods than babies can without teeth. Include children in writing a thank-you note to the visiting parent.

💬 ⚗️ ♥

MATERIALS
- paper and crayons

OTHER IDEAS

- Visit an animal breeder, farm, petting zoo, or pet store to see the mouths of young animals that have not yet grown their teeth. Teach children how to be gentle with the baby animals. Ask the expert to explain to the children what the young animals eat and how their diets will change once they have teeth.

  💬 ⚗️ ♥

- Visit a park or plant nursery to see plant roots, or provide plants with roots for children to plant. Explain to the children why roots are important to plants. Tell them that their teeth have roots too, but the dentist needs special equipment to see them.

  💬 ⚗️

- Take photos of each child's mouth with teeth showing, and write the child's name on the back of the photo. See if children can pick out their own photos. If they need help, provide a nonbreakable mirror. Non-breakable mirrors can also be used for counting their teeth and seeing what their teeth look like. Talk about what teeth and gums look like. Make the camera available for children to take mouth pictures of friends, classroom visitors, and family members.

  💬 ➕ ♥ 🖥️

- With the children, make a list of all the ways teeth can be helpful. Ask questions or give hints if they do not mention the following: taking a bite (of an apple or a sandwich), chewing food once it is in the mouth, making their smiles brighter, helping them speak clearly, and whistling. Encour-age children to illustrate the list, and post it to remind them of the importance of their teeth.

Toothbrush Inspection

Hold up a toothbrush, and ask children to describe what it is and how it is used. Show children more toothbrushes, making sure each one is different from the others because of its size (child or adult), color, shape, type of bristles (soft or medium), type of head (rectangle or oval), age (new or well used), or operation (manual, electric, or battery-operated). Ask children if each item they see is a toothbrush, and then encourage a discussion about how the toothbrushes are alike and how they are different. Count the total number of toothbrushes. Display the variety of toothbrushes so children can handle, examine, and continue discussing the brushes after the activity. Explain that classroom toothbrushes are for everyone to use to learn about toothbrushes, but they are not to be used in anyone's mouth. Tell children they should put only their own toothbrushes into their mouths—no one else's.

MATERIALS
- a variety of toothbrushes, including electric and battery-operated ones

OTHER IDEAS
- Visit a store to see and discuss a wide range of oral-hygiene products, such as floss, water flossers, toothpaste, mouthwash, and whitening strips.

- Let children paint with a variety of brushes. Talk about how there are many kinds of paintbrushes, just as there are many kinds of toothbrushes.

- Play the song "The Pearly White Waltz" by Tickle Tune Typhoon, and move to the rhythm.

- Show children a variety of commercial and homemade toothbrush holders for use at home and at school, and encourage them to compare the holders. Help them see that some holders are for single brushes and others are for more than one brush. Stress the importance of storing individual brushes so they do not touch and can have air around them. Place sample holders where children can practice putting in class toothbrushes (not ones for individuals to use) and taking them out.

Toothbrush Wiggle

Have a small group of children wiggle and jiggle their fingers, toes, arms, legs, heads, and whole bodies. Tell children that when they brush their teeth, they should wiggle and jiggle their toothbrushes on all parts of their teeth. Invite children to show you their upper teeth, lower teeth, biting surfaces, inner surfaces, and outer surfaces. Show children the correct way to brush teeth, and let them practice. Label toothbrushes, and store them in a way that allows plenty of air to circulate around them but doesn't allow them to touch one another.

MATERIALS

■ a toothbrush for each child, a tube of toothpaste for each child, water, and storage containers

OTHER IDEAS

■ Provide dolls or other toys with teeth. Ask children to count the number of teeth each doll has and to practice brushing the doll's teeth using the correct technique.

■ Let children use a nonbreakable mirror to examine their own teeth, count them, and describe what their teeth look like. Encourage them to look at their teeth using a variety of nonbreakable mirrors and holding their mouths in a variety of shapes. Talk about how to hold a toothbrush so that it can reach all parts of all teeth.

■ Encourage children to move their bodies up, down, and around when music is played. Then show them how to move their toothbrushes up, down, and around in a circular motion. Let them practice the toothbrushing movements with imaginary brushes.

■ Play the song "Brush Your Teeth" by Raffi.

Sticky Snack

Introduce the word *sticky,* and let children feel a sticky object, such as tape, to help them understand the concept. Give children a snack that consists of something sticky and something that is not sticky. Ask them which food is sticky and how it feels in their mouths. Help them concentrate on how the sticky element feels, not how it tastes. Explain that sticky foods stick to their teeth and can cause tooth decay if not removed. End the activity by having children brush their teeth to brush off the sticky snack.

❗ Safety Note: Sticky foods, such as peanut butter, marshmallows, and raisins, can block children's air passages. Supervise children closely, and encourage them to take small bites and chew carefully during this activity. Be aware of whether any children have peanut allergies, and use alternative sticky foods as needed for safety.

MATERIALS
- tape or other sticky object, a sticky snack (such as caramel, honey, syrup, raisins, marshmallows, or bread), a nonsticky snack (such as apples or carrots), a toothbrush for each child, a tube of toothpaste for each child, and water

OTHER IDEAS
- Gather a variety of sticky objects (such as tape, an adhesive bandage, contact paper, and glue) and sticky foods (such as honey, syrup, and marshmallows) for children to explore and discuss. Afterward, while children are washing their hands, ask them which things were the easiest and hardest to wash off.

- Provide pictures of sticky and nonsticky food for children to sort.

- Add an assortment of sticky things (such as many kinds of tape, stickers, glitter, and glue) to the art interest area, and as children use the materials, talk informally with them about how sticky food can cause tooth decay if not removed.

- Help children make no-cook sticky glue by adding water to flour until it feels gooey and then tossing in a bit of salt. As children wash their hands to remove the glue, compare their fingers to their teeth, and explain that both have difficult places to clean. Areas around fingernails and between fingers are similar to those around the base of teeth and be-

tween teeth. Use the glue for art projects, such as making a collage of sticky-food pictures.

Doggie Teeth

Arrange for a good-natured dog, one accustomed to young children, to visit the classroom. Prior to the visit, ask children to talk about what they think the dog's teeth and gums will look like and how many teeth the dog will have. Ask them to draw a picture of what the dog's teeth and gums may look like. When the dog arrives, have a few children at a time look closely at its mouth to see its gums and teeth. Encourage them to bring their drawings of dog gums and teeth near the dog so they can see how close their predictions were. After they have seen the real thing, children may be interested in drawing another picture to more accurately reflect the dog's gums and teeth. Ask children if they know what kind of health helper looks at people's teeth as they looked at the dog's teeth. Let them know that the dentist checks our teeth, helps fix teeth that are not healthy, and teaches us how to take better care of our teeth. Involve children in sending a dog bone or biscuit and a thank-you note to the dog and its owner.

❗ Safety Note: Even gentle dogs can become aggressive when frightened. Be sure to prepare children on how to approach the dog. Limit the number of children who can approach the dog at a time, and have an adult overseeing the dog at all times.

MATERIALS
- a gentle dog, art supplies, paper, pencils, and a dog bone

OTHER IDEAS
- Encourage children to look in magazines to find pictures and photographs of people and animals showing their teeth. Guide children in cutting out just the mouths and teeth to glue onto craft sticks. Suggest that children show their teeth pictures to one another. Ask them to guess if the teeth belong to a person or an animal, and then have them guess the age of the person or the kind of animal.

- Add teeth samples, real and replicas, to an area for children to explore and discuss. Large educational models of human teeth and giant toothbrushes are just the beginning. Educational skull models with teeth can help children see the teeth in context. Animal skulls with teeth may be found in the woods and on farmland. Consider showing tooth replicas of dinosaurs, sharks, lions, and other animals of interest to children. Dentists may provide examples of dental moldings.

Real teeth or dentures obtained for the collection can be placed in a clear, locked box for viewing, like at a museum.

💬 ⚗️

■ Show children novelty toys like chattering teeth and costume vampire fangs to get their attention. Encourage a discussion of the similarities and differences between their teeth and the novelty ones.

💬 ⚗️

■ Provide clay or playdough, and encourage each child to create a mouth showing teeth. If none of the children are at the stage where they may try to eat small objects, make available small objects (such as beads, gravel, and beans) that can represent teeth. Film each child showing and telling about the mouth full of teeth she created. Make the video available in the classroom and to families.

🎨 🏃 💻

Breanne Brushes

Involve children in creating and decorating two toothbrushing charts each, one for school and one to take home. Ask children to mark their charts when they brush their teeth at school. Observe to see if they use the appropriate technique and if they brush for a full two minutes. After they brush, show them a doll, and tell them that the doll's name is Breanne. Tell them that Breanne does not want to brush her teeth. Ask them to help Breanne understand why brushing is important. Listen to their reasons to assess their levels of understanding.

MATERIALS

- heavy paper or construction paper, art supplies, rulers, a toothbrush for each child, a tube of toothpaste for each child, water, and a doll

OTHER IDEAS

- Film a group of children demonstrating proper toothbrushing and explaining why toothbrushing is important. Show the video to the class, and make it available in the classroom and to families.

- Explain to children that they should brush their teeth for two minutes. Help them understand how long two minutes is by having them do the following for two minutes: dance to music, listen to a short story, march in place, sing a song, or practice deep-breathing exercises.

- Show children a variety of tools for measuring two minutes: a timer with an audible buzz, a stopwatch, a clock with a second hand, an hourglass sand timer, and a two-minute song. Select one of the tools to use with children as they brush their teeth. Alternate tools over time.

- Encourage children to demonstrate what they know about taking care of their teeth by creating a poem, song, story, or poster to share with the class.

FAMILY INFORMATION

TAKING CARE OF MY SMILE!

All teeth are important, even primary (baby) teeth! Preschoolers usually have twenty teeth. Permanent teeth start to come in when children are about six years old.

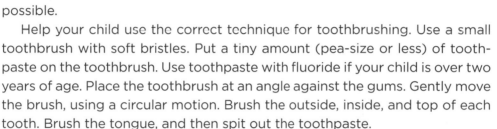

Children should brush their teeth twice each day. The most important time to brush is before going to bed, because bacteria can build up in the mouth overnight if food particles are present. These bacteria can cause tooth decay, gum problems, and bad breath. Children should also brush after breakfast if possible.

Help your child use the correct technique for toothbrushing. Use a small toothbrush with soft bristles. Put a tiny amount (pea-size or less) of toothpaste on the toothbrush. Use toothpaste with fluoride if your child is over two years of age. Place the toothbrush at an angle against the gums. Gently move the brush, using a circular motion. Brush the outside, inside, and top of each tooth. Brush the tongue, and then spit out the toothpaste.

Brush for at least two minutes. Using a timer can help you and your child know when two minutes is over. Your child will need help brushing her or his teeth. As your child learns to brush, check his or her teeth, and help brush any spots she or he missed.

If brushing is not possible, encourage your child to swish and spit with water after eating. This action helps remove food and reduces bacteria in the mouth.

VISIT A DENTIST

Children should visit a dentist at least every six months. Help prepare your child for a visit to the dentist. Most dental clinics have activities to make visits more fun for children. Discuss how dentists and hygienists help take care of teeth. Look at each other's teeth in a mirror, and discuss how dentists use a small mirror to see teeth. Practice opening your mouths to see who can open the widest.

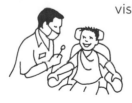

FAMILY ACTIVITY

Glue this picture to one side of an empty cereal box, and then
cut out the puzzle pieces, using the lines as guides. While working the
puzzle with your child, talk about the importance of cleaning our
mouths and teeth and when and how to keep teeth clean.

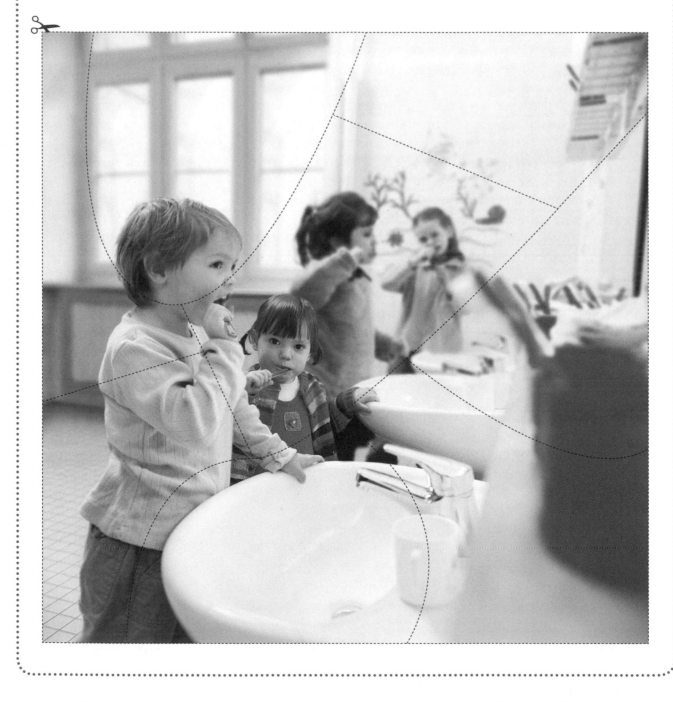

5

Stopping Germs before They Stop Me!

LEARNING OBJECTIVES

- Children will communicate that germs are so tiny they cannot be seen.
- Children will cover their mouths and noses when coughing or sneezing.
- Children will practice hand hygiene, including using the correct hand-washing technique and washing at appropriate times.

Young children are exposed to germs in many ways. They put items into their mouths; they explore their surroundings through touching and then put their fingers into their mouths; and they are close to the dirty ground and floor level. These normal behaviors and circumstances expose children to a multitude of germs. Young children are at higher risk for diseases than adults because their bodies do not have as much resistance to illnesses. Their natural immune systems are still developing, and they may not yet have full immunity to diseases (such as measles and mumps) through immunizations. Proper hand hygiene (such as hand washing and hand sanitizing) helps protect children from communicable diseases. Frequent and proper hand washing removes most harmful germs before they spread to mouths, noses, eyes, or other people.

Adult modeling promotes proper hand washing. Both adults and children should wash their hands at the following times:

- upon arrival, after breaks, and when moving from one classroom to another
- before and after preparing, eating, and handling food or beverages

- before and after water play
- after toileting
- after handling body fluids (such as after wiping noses or treating wounds)
- after handling animals or cleaning up animal waste
- after playing outdoors or in sand
- after cleaning or handling garbage

Frequent and thorough hand washing with running water rinses away germs. Children and adults should use the following method:

1. Wet hands under running water.

2. Apply soap and rub hands together vigorously until a soapy later appears.

3. Continue to rub hands for at least twenty seconds. Rub the palms, backs of hands, and all areas between fingers, around nail beds, and under fingernails.

4. Rinse hands under running water.

5. Dry hands thoroughly with a disposable paper towel, single-use cloth towel, or air dryer.

6. Turn off water taps with a paper towel.

7. If used, dispose of the paper towel in a wastebasket.

If hands are not visibly soiled, the supervised use of alcohol-based hand sanitizers is an alternative to traditional hand washing with soap and water for children over two years of age (and adults). A single pump of an alcohol-based sanitizer should be dispensed. Hands should be rubbed together—distributing sanitizer to all hand and finger surfaces—and permitted to air-dry.

Disease prevention focuses on preventing the spread of all communicable diseases, whether a child or adult has a cold, diarrhea, head lice, or HIV/AIDS. Disease prevention practices include hand washing and taking precautions to avoid contact with blood and other body fluids, including mucus, saliva, urine, feces, and vomit. Adults should wear disposable nonporous gloves when assisting children in the bathroom, diapering, cleaning up blood or body fluids, and picking up and disposing of trash. Gloves should be worn only once, and hands should be washed after gloves are removed.

Teach children to avoid touching blood and body fluids, and help them understand that germs can be carried through these fluids. Children are better able to understand these procedures when they are related to common diseases with which they are familiar, such as colds.

The Centers for Disease Control and Prevention state that hand washing is the single most effective way to prevent the transmission of diseases. Helping children to follow Henry the Hand's four principles of hand awareness (found at www.henrythehand.com) will greatly reduce the spread of diseases. These four simple directions have been endorsed by the American Medical Association and the American Academy of Family Practitioners:

1. Wash your hands when they are dirty and before eating.

2. Do not cough into your hands.

3. Do not sneeze into your hands.

4. Above all, do not put your fingers into your eyes, nose, or mouth.

VOCABULARY

between	disinfect	rinse	spread
condition	exposure	rub	trash can
contagious	germ	sanitize	virus
contamination	ill	scrub	visible
cough	invisible	sick	
cover	lather	sneeze	
disease	prevent	spray	

CREATING THE ENVIRONMENT

■ The ideal environment includes a sink with warm, running water; liquid soap; paper towels; and a wastebasket within children's reach. (Antibacterial soap is not necessary.)

■ A child's skin is tenderer than an adult's. Water that feels warm to an adult will likely feel hot to a child. Even a brief exposure to hot water can cause second- and third-degree burns. The temperature of hot water should not exceed 120 degrees Fahrenheit (49 degrees Celsius). The water temperature can be controlled either by adjusting the water heater or by installing a temperature regulator. Encourage children to use hot and cold water together to carefully regulate water temperature.

■ Have children create or download hand-washing signs (such as the one found at www.childhealthonline.org); post the signs in relevant classroom areas, such as near the water table, snack area, and sinks.

■ Clean objects and surfaces with soap and water frequently. Cleaning physically removes all dirt and contamination; the friction of cleaning removes most germs.

■ When necessary, sanitize or disinfect objects and surfaces. Sanitizing reduces germs to a level considered safe; disinfecting destroys or inactivates most germs.

■ A bleach and water solution of one-fourth cup of regular bleach to one gallon of water—or one tablespoon of bleach to one quart of water—is an effective and inexpensive general sanitizer. Areas soiled with blood or body fluids can be disinfected with a solution of one-fourth cup of bleach to one quart of water. Solutions must be made daily because the solution's effectiveness diminishes over time. Keep bleach and unused solution in a locked cabinet or closet. Because purchased bleach concentrations may vary, check with your local health department or child care health consultant for specific ratios of bleach to water.

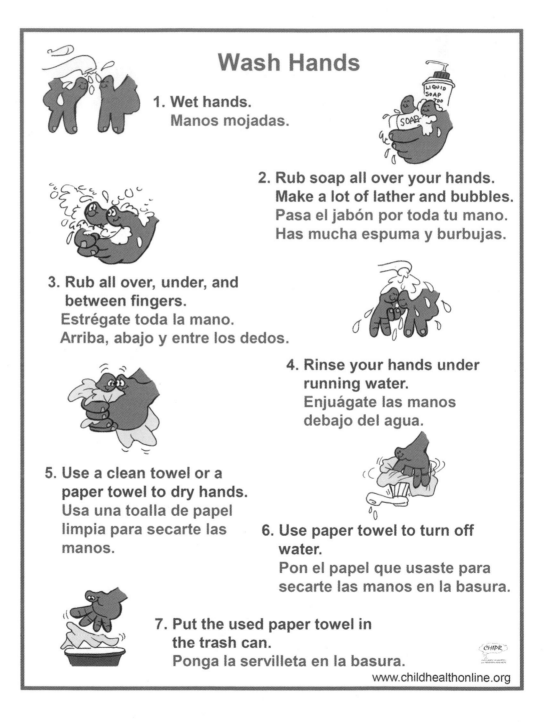

Wash Hands

1. **Wet hands.**
   Manos mojadas.

2. **Rub soap all over your hands.**
   Make a lot of lather and bubbles.
   Pasa el jabón por toda tu mano.
   Has mucha espuma y burbujas.

3. **Rub all over, under, and between fingers.**
   Estrégate toda la mano.
   Arriba, abajo y entre los dedos.

4. **Rinse your hands under running water.**
   Enjuágate las manos debajo del agua.

5. **Use a clean towel or a paper towel to dry hands.**
   Usa una toalla de papel limpia para secarte las manos.

6. **Use paper towel to turn off water.**
   Pon el papel que usaste para secarte las manos en la basura.

7. **Put the used paper towel in the trash can.**
   Ponga la servilleta en la basura.

CHIPR

www.childhealthonline.org

EVALUATION

- During role playing, do children talk about or show how to avoid germs?

- Are children increasingly covering their mouths and noses when coughing or sneezing (using the elbow or tissue method)?

- Do children increasingly wash their hands correctly?

- Do children ask about or initiate hand washing at appropriate times?

- Do children communicate their ideas about what germs might look like if they could see them?

CHILDREN'S ACTIVITIES

The Disappearing Act

Invite a professional or amateur magician to perform for children, or show a video of magic being performed. Help children learn about the concepts of invisibility and being out of sight by watching things disappear during the show. Tell children that germs, which are tiny little creatures that live everywhere, are also invisible unless you look for them with special equipment. Let them know that some germs do not harm us, but some can make us sick. Let them know they are going to be learning more about germs and how to get rid of them. With the magician's approval, invite a local television station or newspaper to visit and report on the magic show and the children's study of germs. Remember to also obtain parent permission to include children's images or names in the media, including social media, such as Facebook.

MATERIALS

- materials requested by the magician (if any) or a video of magic being performed

OTHER IDEAS

- Perform a few magic tricks for the children, and then teach them to the children.

- Play hide-and-seek with objects, and talk about how the objects are still there even though the children can't see them, just as germs are still there even though the children can't see them. Give children a chance to hide objects for one another to find.

- Play hide-and-seek with the children, and discuss how they don't really disappear when hiding but are out of sight, just as germs are out of sight.

- Make crayon etchings by encouraging children to use crayons to fill a sheet of card stock with bright colors. Encourage children to fill all spaces on the paper with color. Let children use black tempera paint or black crayons to rub over the entire page, covering up all of the color. After the paint dries, give children craft sticks or other objects for drawing a picture, lines, or shapes through the black paint so the background color shows. Remind children that the original colors were always there but could not be seen under the black paint or crayon. Compare this concept to germs.

Invisible Germs

Because germs are not visible to the naked eye, most young children will develop only a minimal understanding about them, but you can still introduce the concept. Take care not to frighten children about germs. Read *Those Mean Nasty Dirty Downright Disgusting but . . . Invisible Germs/Esos Desagradables Detestables Sucios Completamente Asquerosos pero . . . Invisibles Gérmenes* by Judith Anne Rice. Encourage children to talk about the book and to ask questions. Point out that not everyone who is sick is contagious and that some diseases are not transmittable. Keep a list of the questions so you can help children find the answers. Tell them you will look for resource books and experts to help with their questions. Make sure to follow through.

MATERIALS

- a copy of *Those Mean Nasty Dirty Downright Disgusting but . . . Invisible Germs / Esos Desagradables Detestables Sucios Completamente Asquerosos pero . . . Invisibles Gérmenes* by Judith Anne Rice, paper, and a marker

OTHER IDEAS

- Let children talk about people they know who are sick, and let them know that some people who are sick are not contagious.

- Invite someone who has a noncontagious disease or condition to visit and talk about the disease or condition.

- Arrange to visit a high school, college, or community science lab to learn about germs by talking with experts (such as teachers or doctors) and looking through microscopes at germs. Help children formulate questions in advance.

- Invite a medical professional or scientist to visit the classroom and talk about germs.

Hands of Friends

Encourage children to examine their hands to see their unique characteristics. Have them look for differences in palm lines and fingerprint lines. Point out and discuss any moles, freckles, calluses, wrinkles, scars, or other distinguishing marks. Explain that we can show our hands to someone else to examine, but we should not touch anyone unless that person says it is okay. Ask children if they want to show their hands to a classmate. Help children compare the sizes, shapes, and colors of their hands. Tell children to compare their fingernails to other fingernails to see how they are alike and different. Provide magnifying glasses and measuring instruments. Ask children to name what they have touched with their hands today (such as toys, forks, books, the floor, and handrails). Let children know that clean hands are an important part of being healthy and that they should wash their hands often because they touch so many things that have germs on them.

MATERIALS
- magnifying glasses, rulers, and tape measures

OTHER IDEAS
- Photocopy and display pictures of children's hands in a variety of positions (such as palms up, palms down, folded, and in a fist). See if children can identify their own hands.

- Let children make model hands using materials they identify, such as clay, cloth, or paper.

- Encourage children to paint their hands using washable liquid tempera paint and to make handprints on paper. Encourage children to compare their handprints. Let them wash their hands until all of the paint is removed, and discuss the places where the paint was the most difficult to remove.

- Visit a store to see mannequin hands, or visit a museum or art store to see pictures and sculptures of hands.

Hand-Washing Interviews

Tell children that they will interview people about hand washing. Encourage them to think of questions. List their questions on a piece of paper, and add to the list as children think of others. Arrange a time for adults to be interviewed by one small group of children at a time. Select people who wash their hands because of their jobs, such as nurses, doctors, preschool teachers, cooks, food servers, janitors, artists, sanitation workers, dentists, and mechanics. Interviewees could be family members of the children or employees of the program. Take children on a field trip to conduct their interviews, or invite guests to the classroom. Give each small group a chance to report to another group about the interview. With permission of the interviewees, film the interview and make the video available for children to review.

MATERIALS

■ paper, marker, a video camera, and a viewing device for the video

OTHER IDEAS

■ Go for a walk to look for posted signs throughout the building and beyond about hand washing.

■ Visit a physical therapist or invite one to the classroom, and learn about hand exercises and related tools. Practice exercises with children.

■ Visit a doctor to see pictures and models of hands to learn about the bones, muscles, tendons, joints, ligaments, and cartilage in hands.

■ Visit a salon so children can watch how fingernails are manicured, or invite a professional to visit the classroom to demonstrate how to care for nails.

❶ Safety Note: Be aware that nail salons may have noxious odors due to harsh nail chemicals, especially later in the day. Consider the ventilation of the salon. Hair salons that also provide manicures may have fewer odors.

Lather Up

In small groups, show children the correct hand-washing procedure, and encourage them to practice the following:

1. Wet hands under running water and apply soap.

2. Rub hands together vigorously until a soapy lather appears; then continue to rub them for at least twenty seconds. Rub the palms, backs of hands, and all areas between fingers, around nail beds, and under fingernails.

3. Rinse hands under running water.

4. Dry hands thoroughly with a disposable paper towel, single-use cloth towel, or air dryer.

5. Turn off water taps with a paper towel.

6. If used, dispose of paper towel in the wastebasket.

MATERIALS
- warm running water, liquid soap, clean paper towels, and a wastebasket or air dryer

OTHER IDEAS

- Involve children in making and illustrating signs that remind them to wash their hands before they eat, after they paint, after they go to the bathroom, after they blow their noses, before and after they play in sand or water, and whenever their hands are dirty.

- While children are washing their hands, ask them where they think the water goes when it goes down the drain. Help them investigate this question if they show interest.

- Visit a construction site to see a building's plumbing system, or invite a plumber to visit, show pipes, and talk about her job.

- Read and discuss books like *You Are Healthy* by Todd Snow and *Germs Are Not for Sharing* by Elizabeth Verdick.

Secret Spray

Let children spray lemon juice on a sheet of paper, and draw their attention to how the spray barely shows up. After the paper dries, use heat to make the spray visible—for example, by holding the paper near a lightbulb, placing it under a heating pad, ironing it without steam, placing it in a warm oven for about ten minutes, or leaving it in the hot sun. Tell children that when they cough or sneeze, they spray invisible germs, just like they sprayed lemon juice on the paper. Show them how to turn away from others when they cough or sneeze and how to cover their coughs or sneezes with tissues or their elbows. Stress the importance of washing their hands afterward.

❗ Safety Note: Use caution when operating an iron or oven with children nearby. Be sure adequate supervision is available, and never leave the appliance unattended.

MATERIALS
- lemon juice, spray bottles, paper, and a heat source (such as a lightbulb, heating pad, iron, oven, or the sun)

OTHER IDEAS
- Ask children to describe times when they sneezed or coughed. Prompt them with questions to encourage details.

- Involve children in mixing baking soda and water in equal parts and using a funnel to pour the liquid into a spray bottle. Let children spray the mixture onto paper. Let the paper dry, and then either hold the paper to a warm nonhalogen lightbulb or paint the paper with grape juice to reveal the sprayed picture. Remind children that invisible germs spray from their noses and mouths when they sneeze.

- Mix tempera paint to a thin consistency, and pour it into spray bottles. Let children spray designs onto cardboard boxes or other surfaces using a variety of paint colors. Remind them that invisible germs spray from their noses and mouths when they sneeze.

- Let children use spray bottles filled with water in the outdoors. Suggest that they mist plants to give them a drink, create water pictures on solid fences or sidewalks, or even mist visible parts of their bodies to cool down.

FAMILY INFORMATION

STOPPING GERMS BEFORE THEY STOP ME!

Children share germs in many ways. They put their fingers in their mouths, they explore their surroundings through touching, and their toileting and hygiene habits are not well developed. Most diseases are spread when children (and adults) touch their faces, eyes, noses, and mouths. Washing hands is the best way to prevent the spread of germs!

Using soap and running water is the best way to wash hands. Show your child how to make soap bubbles and how to rub the bubbles all over his or her hands and wrists and between fingers. Make sure your child checks for dirt under the fingernails too. Rub the bubbles for at least twenty seconds. This is about how long it takes to sing "The Alphabet Song." Rinse your child's hands with running water. Dry hands with a clean towel or a disposable paper towel.

HAND SANITIZER

For children over two years of age, alcohol-based hand sanitizer can be used. A single pump of the sanitizer is enough. Rub the sanitizer all over the hands and between fingers. Waving hands in the air to dry them is a fun option!

Supervise your child when she or he uses hand sanitizer. Many of these products smell like fruit or candy, but they can be toxic if swallowed. Keep the hand sanitizer in its original container and out of your child's reach.

FAMILY ACTIVITY

Attach this sheet to cardboard. Cut out game pieces and players. Each person playing should choose a player. Put game pieces in a small container. Take turns drawing out a game piece to see how to move each player along the board. If the player lands on a space with a picture, use the key to see what should happen. After a move is completed, return the game piece to the container. The first player to reach the "Finish" space wins. Use this game to initiate a discussion about how germs cause many illnesses and about how cleanliness helps prevent illness.

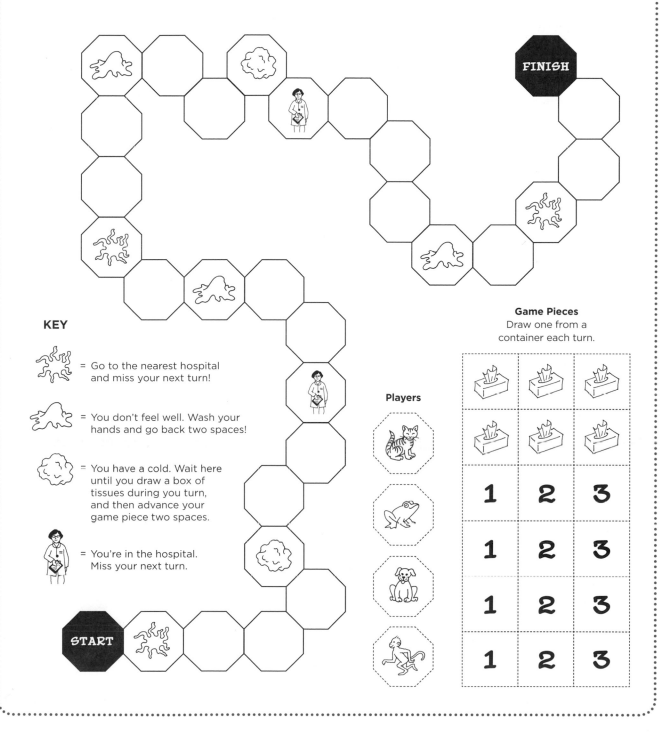

KEY

= Go to the nearest hospital and miss your next turn!

= You don't feel well. Wash your hands and go back two spaces!

= You have a cold. Wait here until you draw a box of tissues during you turn, and then advance your game piece two spaces.

= You're in the hospital. Miss your next turn.

Players

Game Pieces
Draw one from a container each turn.

1	2	3
1	2	3
1	2	3
1	2	3

My Medicine Is for Me!

LEARNING OBJECTIVES

- Children will state that it is appropriate to take medicine when sick and to prevent diseases.

- Children will identify individuals who can give them medicine.

- Children will communicate that medicine comes in many forms (for example, in pills, liquids, and shots).

Medicines can be crucial to the health and wellness of children, but both prescription medications and over-the-counter products (such as acetaminophen, ibuprofen, and allergy medications) can be dangerous if given incorrectly. Keep all medicines in their original labeled containers, and store them in locked cabinets that are inaccessible to children. As much as possible, avoid giving medication in the early childhood or school setting. When possible, parents and guardians should give medicine at home.

Family beliefs and practices regarding the use of medicine and the procedure for administering it may vary. For example, some families rarely use either prescription or OTC medications; other families may give a daily vitamin to their children. At enrollment, gather information from families about their practices so you can teach children and provide support and resources appropriate to their individual situations.

Family practices may also vary in who is allowed to give medicine to children. Parents, grandparents, or older siblings may assist children with medication. Some children may self-administer specific medications, such as an asthma inhaler. Help children understand that each medication has a specific purpose and should only be taken when needed. Medicine is not candy, and taking medicine is not a play activity.

Some children are exposed to drug misuse and abuse in their homes or communities; even so, presenting to young children information on illegal drug use or drug abuse is not appropriate. Instead, present information about when to take medicine and from whom to accept medicine.

In schools and early childhood programs, only designated and trained staff members should administer medication to children. Program policies on administering medication should be clearly written and include guidelines on who can give medicine at school, what paperwork is required prior to administration of medicine, where medicine should be stored, and what documentation is necessary after administration. Ask about the possible side effects of medication given to children in your class, and be prepared to deal with those noted.

The five "rights" of medication administration are: (1) the right child, (2) the right medication, (3) the right time, (4) the right dose, and (5) the right route (for example, oral or topical). A sixth requirement is to complete the right documentation.

VOCABULARY

botany	fever	lotion	sting
broken	hurt	pharmacist	syringe
capsule	immunization	pill	tablet
cream	injection	prescription	vitamins
directions	itch	scratch	
dose	label	shot	
eyedropper	liquid	sick	

CREATING THE ENVIRONMENT

- Keep medicines in their original labeled containers, and store them as directed (for example, some medicines require refrigeration) in locked cabinets or boxes that are inaccessible to children.

- Provide many types of clean and empty medicine containers for children to see as they learn about taking or applying medicines. Include pillboxes and pill bottles, cream and lotion boxes and bottles, spray bottles, and new unused syringes without needles.

EVALUATION

- Do children discuss who does or can give them medicine?
- During role playing, do children communicate the appropriate situations for taking medicine?
- Can children identify pills, shots, and other items as medicine?
- Can children communicate why a doctor might give them medicine?
- Do children state why they should not take medicine without permission?

CHILDREN'S ACTIVITIES

Pills and Potions

Show children empty and clean medicine containers or photographs of medicine containers for common over-the-counter medicines for children. Ask children if they recognize the containers and can tell you about them. Encourage children to talk about experiences they have had with medicine, including why they needed medicine and who gave it to them. On a large sheet of paper, write down the key information children describe as they recount their experiences with medicine, including who gave each child medicine.

💬 ❤️

❗ Safety Note: Be sure containers are empty and clean.

MATERIALS
- empty and clean containers of common medicines for children (including containers for pills, liquids, and creams) or mounted pictures of common medicines for children (including children's vitamins and medicines for coughing, fevers, itching, scratches, bites, and stings), chart paper, and a marker

OTHER IDEAS
- Play the song "98.8" by Justin Roberts, and listen to the words. Talk about how important it is for children to let an adult know when they feel sick and how important it is to tell the truth about feeling sick so they can get the right medicine.
🎨 💬 ⚗️

- Assist each child in making a book that shows pictures (such as drawings, photographs, or magazine advertisements) of medicines or natural remedies (such as ice) they have used. Include the names or pictures of the adults who gave them the medicine or remedy. Offer to print captions in the books for children who are not yet writing.
🎨 💬 💻

- Show children pictures of medicine cabinets, and ask if they have seen anything like them. Explain that medicine cabinets are frequently found in bathrooms of homes. Tell children that medicine cabinets are not the only place where medicine is stored. Ask if they know of other places for storing medicine. See if they know where medicine is kept at school. Show children where medicine is locked up, and explain who is allowed to get the medicine and give it to children. Help them understand that locking up medicine and limiting the people who have access to it is for their safety.

💬 💻

■ Visit a home supply store so children can see a variety of medicine cabinets, or provide a medicine cabinet in the classroom for children to examine. Let each child create a medicine cabinet display by gluing empty, clean medicine containers inside a small box (such as a shoe box) and decorating the box. Encourage children to talk about who has access to their medicine cabinet and why.

🎨 💬 🏃 ❤️

A Close Look

Provide a labeled display showing a variety of medicine containers, pictures of medicine, vitamins glued to cards and laminated, and dispensing tools. Invite children to examine the medicine display and to talk about what they see. Help them identify the ways medicine can look (for example, a liquid, a capsule, and chewable and nonchewable tablets). Point out that medicine is not candy, even though some pills may look like it. Help them see the various ways medicine can be taken (such as by injecting, receiving drops, chewing, swallowing, and drinking). Show children a container with a prescription label. Explain that some medicine can be purchased by adults without a doctor's approval, whereas other medicine must be purchased from a pharmacist—a special health care professional—and with a doctor's prescription. Remind children that they should take medicine only if their parents or guardians tell them it is all right to do so.

💬 💻

❗ Safety Note: Be sure containers are empty and clean. Do not leave pills used for display unattended. After the activity, remove the pills from the display. Even dietary supplements, like iron tablets, can be toxic for young children.

MATERIALS
■ empty and clean prescription and over-the-counter medicine containers (including containers for sprays, liquids, and creams and one with an eye-dropper), pictures of medicine, vitamins glued to cards and laminated, and a variety of dispensing tools (including new unused syringes without needles, medicine spoons, and medicine cups)

OTHER IDEAS
■ Visit a pharmacy, or invite a pharmacist to visit the classroom to talk about his job, the tools he uses, and the many kinds of medicine he dispenses. Visit an animal clinic, or invite a veterinarian to display and talk about medicine for animals.
💬 🧪 💻

■ Add empty medicine boxes to the art interest area so children can cut them into pieces to make jigsaw puzzles.
🎨 🏃

■ Play the song "Sign My Cast" by Justin Roberts, and listen to the words. Have children make casts for classroom dolls or toy people using papier-mâché (which requires flour, water, and newspaper strips).
🎨 🏃 🧪

■ Provide new unused syringes without needles, eyedroppers, medicine spoons, medicine cups, and other medicine containers. Encourage children to use these dispensers to practice measuring colored water. Have children compare the amount of water each dispenser holds.

Now and Then

Show children a variety of containers for children's vitamins, and ask if they know what kind of medicine the containers hold and when the medicine should be taken. Explain to children that sometimes we take medicine (such as vitamins and immunizations) to help us stay healthy and sometimes we take medicine to help us get well and feel better when we are sick. Let children talk about their experiences with taking vitamins and getting immunizations to stay healthy and with taking medicine to get well.

MATERIALS

- empty and clean children's vitamin containers

OTHER IDEAS

- Play the song "Doctor, Doctor" by Justin Roberts, and listen to the words. Invite a doctor or nurse to talk with the children about when to take medicine and why taking just the right amount is important.

- Invite family members to talk about the over-the-counter and prescribed medicines (or natural remedies) their family members use. Ask guests to talk about what the medicines look like, how often they take them, and why they take them.

- Read a book about going to the doctor, such as *Froggy Goes to the Doctor* by Jonathan London, and discuss vaccines and other reasons people see a doctor.

- Read a book about an itch, such as *Big Smelly Bear* by Britta Teckentrup or *Rhino's Great Big Itch!* by Natalie Chivers. Explain to children that sometimes an itch can be taken care of without medicine, but other times topical medicine is needed.

Botany

Introduce the word *botany* to children, and explain that it is the study of plants. Ask children if they have any ideas about why people would study plants. Possible reasons might be that some plants are used in medicine and that some plants are used for visual pleasure, food, fuel, building supplies, and clothing. Show them an aloe vera plant, and explain how its leaves can be opened and softly rubbed on the skin to soothe burns. Let them gently feel the plant inside and out. Tell children that although some plants are used for food and medicine, knowing which plants are used for which purpose is hard. Explain that some plants are poisonous. Tell children they should never taste a plant or its seeds or berries unless they ask an adult first. Remind them that they should always wash their hands after touching plants. Invite children to go outside and examine some plants; encourage them to look in a plant guidebook to identify the plants.

❗ Safety Note: Warn children that aloe vera is not safe to eat, and tell them not to taste the plant. Supervise children and make sure they wash their hands after the activity. Remove the plant after the activity.

MATERIALS
- an aloe vera plant and field guides of area plants

OTHER IDEAS

- Visit a nature preserve, and take a guided tour. Ask the guide to point out any plants used for medicine and to explain their importance.

- Invite a professional herbalist to show children herbal products (such as tablets, capsules, powders, teas, and dried plants) and tools (such as a mortar and pestle). Ask the visitor to demonstrate how to process a live plant and to explain how herbs can be used for dietary supplements.

- Visit or grow an herb garden, and explore with children how herbs can be used for medicine. Encourage children to rub plants between their fingers and to smell and taste fresh herbs.

- Gather leaves of herbs to press between waxed paper, blotting paper, the pages of books, or bricks to preserve them. Observe and discuss changes in the leaves over time.

The Natural Way

Show children a display of natural remedies, and ask what they can tell you about them. Explain that some people use natural remedies—such as heat, ice, and certain foods—instead of medicine. Tell them that some people use honey for sore throats, bee stings, or dry skin. Tell them that baking soda may be used to ease itching. Let them mix three tablespoons of baking soda into a baby bathtub or dishpan that is half full of water. Have them give an itch-soothing bath to a baby doll. Remind children to let an adult know if they are hurt or think they need medicine.

MATERIALS

- several kinds of ice packs, ice, several kinds of heating pads, a hot-water bottle, a humidifier, honey, baking soda, a washable doll, a baby bathtub or dishpan, and clean water

OTHER IDEAS

- Invite children's family members to show and tell about the natural remedies they use in their family.

- Read *A Sick Day for Amos McGee* by Philip C. Stead, and discuss the ways friends helped in the story.

- Help children identify ways to apply cold without using a commercial ice pack. Provide children with washcloths, and let them dip the cloths in water, wring them out, and put them in freezer bags with their names on them. Place the bags in a freezer until the next day. When children remove the cloths from the bags, encourage them to place the cold cloths on parts of their bodies (such as knees, elbows, and ankles) to see how the cold feels.

- Fill a hot-water bottle with hot water, and let children feel it. Discuss ways heat can be used to help people feel better. Place the hot-water bottle by a clock. Every five minutes, ask a few children to check the hot-water bottle to see if it is still warm. On chart paper, assist them (as needed) in marking the time they checked the bottle, the agreed upon yes or no decision regarding the heat, and their initials. Once a small group of children make the decision that the hot-water bottle is no longer warm, call all children together so that the small group can report their findings. Let children know how long the hot-water bottle stayed warm.

Artistic Messages

Review with children what they have learned about medicines. Write on a large sheet of paper the primary messages you want them to remember. Primary medicine messages may include these:

- Some medicines keep us from getting sick.

- Some medicines help us get well or feel better.

- Medicine should be given only by the people parents or guardians allow.

- Medicine is not candy.

- Medicine comes in many forms, such as in pills, liquids, sprays, and creams.

- Sometimes remedies other than medicine can help us feel better when we are sick or hurt.

Encourage each child to pick one of the main messages and to make an illustrated poster with the message on it. Have children copy the message onto their poster, write out the message for them, or type up the message on a computer and print out multiple copies for children to use.

MATERIALS
- a large sheet of paper, a marker, and art supplies

OTHER IDEAS

- After reading and discussing the directions on empty and clean medicine containers, help children decorate the containers to make vases. Decorating might include painting the containers, gluing twigs all the way around, painting the containers with glue and dipping them in sand, attaching small pieces of overlapping masking tape or duct tape to cover the total surface, gluing sequins on the container, or any other creative technique.

- Encourage children to use clay or modeling clay to make "pills." Ask children to count the pills, explain what they are for, tell you the proper dosage, and describe where they should be stored. Let children take pictures of their pills before cleanup time.

- Using empty and clean medicine containers, help children create musical instruments. Pebbles or jingle bells can be put into the containers for shaking. Lidless plastic bottles can be blown across for whistling. Sandpaper can be glued to two hand-size containers for rubbing together. And rubber bands can be stretched across a box opening for strumming. Challenge children to come up with other musical instruments to make. Once their instruments have been made, help them play the instruments in the background as you read the primary medicine messages.

- Using available materials, such as old socks or paper bags, help each child create a puppet. Once every child has a puppet, use a teacher puppet to initiate a conversation with each child's puppet. Ask questions to see if the child knows the primary medicine messages.

FAMILY INFORMATION

MY MEDICINE IS FOR ME!

When your child needs medicine, you may need to purchase a prescription medicine, such as an antibiotic, from a pharmacist. In other cases, an over-the-counter medicine, such as acetaminophen or a medicine to settle the stomach, is appropriate. You can buy these medicines without a doctor's pre-scription. All medicines are strong. Taking more than one kind of medicine or too much of a single medication can be dangerous. Ask your doctor or pharmacist questions before giving medicine to your child:

- What is the name of the medicine?

- Does it need to be kept in the refrigerator?

- How much should I give my child in each dose? When should I give it?

- Will this medicine cause a stomachache, diarrhea, or drowsiness?

- How will I know if the medicine is working?

- Does my child need to take all the medicine? How many days should I give this medicine?

KEEP MEDICINE OUT OF SIGHT AND OUT OF REACH

Explain to your child that medicine comes in pills, liquids, shots, nose sprays, drops (for ears or eyes), and creams for skin. Talk with your child about who can give him or her medicine and explain why he or she is taking the med-icine. Explain that you may give medicine when she or he is sick. Your child should not get medicine on his or her own. Your child should not take medi-cine from other children.

Always keep medicine in the bottle it came in. Medicine bottles have a child-resistant cap. Keep medicine out of children's reach. A locked cabinet or closet is the safest option.

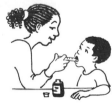

FAMILY ACTIVITY

Assist your child in identifying someone from the following pictures who might be a parent or adult family member (mom, dad, aunt, uncle, and so on), a dentist, and a doctor. Also help in identifying various types of medicine found in the pictures, such as pills, creams, cough syrups, vitamins, and shots or syringes. Talk with your child about who can give her or him medicine and why.

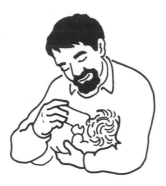 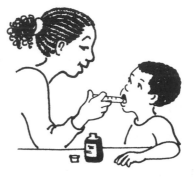

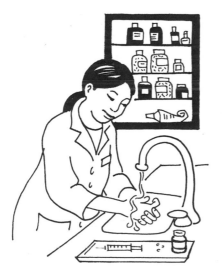 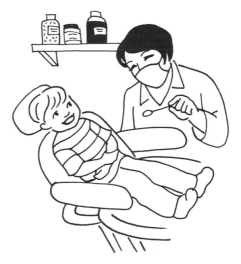